RELAXATION

FOR

CONCENTRATION,

STRESS MANAGEMENT

AND

PAIN CONTROL

~~~ Method

RELAXATION FOR CONCENTRATION, STRESS MANAGEMENT AND PAIN CONTROL
Using the Fleming Method

Edited, and with additional material, by
Carol Horrigan
MSc, SRN, DipN, PGCEA, RCNT, RNT
Nurse Consultant in Complementary Therapies; formerly Lecturer in
Complementary Therapies at The Institute of Advanced Nurse Education,
Royal College of Nursing, London

From the work of Ursula Fleming, compiled by
Anne Fleming
MA (Oxon)

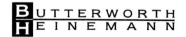

BUTTERWORTH
HEINEMANN

Butterworth-Heinemann
Linacre House, Jordan Hill, Oxford OX2 8DP
A division of Reed Educational and Professional Publishing Ltd

A member of the Reed Elsevier plc group

OXFORD   BOSTON   JOHANNESBURG
MELBOURNE   NEW DELHI   SINGAPORE

First published 1997

British Library Cataloguing in Publication Data
Relaxation for concentration, stress management and pain
  control: using the Fleming method
  1.   Relaxation   2.   Stress management
  I.   Horrigan, Carol   II.   Fleming, Anne
  613.7'9

ISBN 0 7506 2439 6

Typeset by Keyword Typesetting Services Ltd, Wallington and Gt Yarmouth
Printed and bound in Great Britain by Biddles Ltd, Guildford and King's Lynn

Contents

Acknowledgements

There are many people to whom we owe a debt of thanks for their help and without whom this project would not have been possible.

To Lord Craigmyle for his encouragement and support, first of all to Ursula and then to us. To Ursula's children, especially Rory to whom she entrusted her work. To our own families, who helped in so many ways, and to the patients, nurses, relatives and friends who tried the method and gave us the positive feedback that we needed.

Anne Fleming and Carol Horrigan

Foreword

by Anne Fleming

In January 1992, in response to requests from doctors, nurses and physiotherapists, a training centre for instruction in the Fleming Method of relaxation and pain control was set up in Wonersh, Surrey under the auspices of the Albertus Magnus Trust. The centre never opened. Ursula Fleming was admitted to hospital on the day of her first consultation there and she died in March 1992.

Having attended most of Ursula's courses and many of her seminars over the last twenty years, taking part in the lessons and helping to compose explanations of the method, I decided to work on her papers to produce a book for a medical publisher which could serve as a manual for prospective teachers and users of the method. This comprised introductory material, a series of lessons based on transcripts of lessons Ursula gave and some case histories describing her use of the method with terminally ill patients in hospitals and hospices.

Butterworth-Heinemann then invited Carol Horrigan, an experienced nurse educator who had been teaching methods of relaxation and other complementary therapies for many years, to act as editor for the book. She has adapted the lessons for teaching, included discussion of relevant research with references to the literature, and added invaluable advice relating practice of the method to modern medical and nursing procedures.

Even more significantly, she perceived *at first sight* (almost unheard of in Ursula's experience) that the method is unique and judged it so important that she is already training groups of nurses in the UK and will be taking the method to Australia in 1996. By adding to the book a series of her own cases in which she tested the method she has produced further evidence of its efficacy with patients suffering from widely differing conditions.

I am extremely grateful to her. My sister feared the work would die with her: now, through this book, it will go on.

Editor's Preface

I had been using, teaching and researching relaxation methods for more than thirty years when Butterworth-Heinemann asked me if I would edit the book Anne Fleming had compiled from her sister's papers. Her intention was to make the Fleming Method available for doctors and nurses (many of whom had already planned to attend courses at the training centre that Ursula Fleming had set up).

As I read through the text and the hundreds of letters of appreciation Ursula Fleming had received, I realized that she had developed a method of relaxation that was the most uncomplicated I had ever encountered and yet was effective in a wide range of applications because of the common-sense explanations she used to guide the patient through the technique. The simplicity of the method, and the ease with which it can be learned, belies its efficacy, but it is precisely the combination of all these factors which make it ideal for health case practitioners to use within their care programmes, or for individual use by anyone who needs to learn a relaxation technique. The fourteen lessons presented in this book have been compiled from the original teaching and writings of Ursula Fleming and are set out, as far as possible, as she intended – that is, in a 'user-friendly' format. The lesson 'scripts' can be used as they are by the newcomer to relaxation techniques, or amended if circumstances require. They are easily adapted to specific patient needs, and guidelines are included for many of the health problem situations that may make this necessary.

The evidence of several research studies, carried out in different hospitals, testifies to Ursula's commitment to her therapy. That one of these studies was published in *The Practitioner* (Fleming, 1985) was a great accolade, for although the research was carried out in association with doctors and psychologists, as you will read later, Ursula herself had no formal medical training.

This present compilation of her writing and work contains references to research conducted since she published an account for lay people of her relaxation method in her book *Grasping the Nettle: a Positive Approach to Pain*. Many books, research papers and other publications on the practice and efficacy of relaxation methods have subsequently appeared, often containing similarities to Ursula Fleming's earlier book. This may be due to the fact that all relaxation techniques have a common purpose and outcome, and do often display similarities in technique (Kokozka, 1992). They all add weight to the proposal that relaxation as a method of helping reduce symptoms and bring control into patients' lifestyle is a valid adjunct to care. That said, however, there are also many unique, and even startling ideas in the method presented here. Some I have never encountered before and cannot find reference to in any other method, while others are derived from ancient and traditional teachings. Some may even seem extreme to anyone who has used only guided imagery or hypnosis. Brought together as they are in Ursula Fleming's work, they can only reveal the depth of her understanding, the breadth of application of her method (as revealed in the case histories section), and yet the simplicity of its implementation.

What Ursula achieved was years ahead of its time for the majority of health care practitioners working in orthodox settings, where the emphasis has tended to be on developing technological advances in care. She had learned from her own tutor the best of the ancient techniques of relaxation from both Eastern and Western cultures (Hillhouse and Adler, 1991), and some outstandingly different approaches and experiences to benefit patients who are in pain or who may expect it in the course of their illness. Together with her unique philosophical approach to pain, the method offers a positively helpful technique for relaxation which can be used by almost anyone.

Criticisms levelled at other relaxation techniques include the need to be lying down, the need to visualize complicated imaginary scenes suggested by the therapist, or the need to achieve an altered state of consciousness. None of these is required by the Fleming Method, and it can therefore be used by anyone who can understand and hear the instructions of the method. This is particularly important for those members of certain religious groups who may not participate in any altered states of consciousness except under the guidance of their own religious leaders.

The method is initially learnt lying down, if possible, but relaxation can be achieved sitting in a chair or in any other position that the student may have to adopt. Ursula Fleming worked throughout her life towards setting up a school where she could teach her method to any health care worker who wanted to learn. She hoped as many people as possible would learn about relaxation, not just when they were already in pain, but so that they could use it as an everyday part of their lives. When she died prematurely in 1992, with her school just about to open, her hopes could have died with her, but the painstaking compilation of her papers by her sister Anne has made possible the publication of this unique material. Through publishing this book, and setting up workshops and university courses, those hopes may now become a reality.

Carol Horrigan, 1996

Historical background to the Fleming Method

Ursula Fleming was born in Liverpool in 1930, the youngest daughter of two doctors. She was a gifted pianist, and first investigated the use of relaxation to help her with concert performances. She was so impressed with the results of her training by the German relaxation therapist Gertrude Heller that, in the late 1940s, she decided to abandon her musical career and devote herself to the study of relaxation instead.

Mrs Heller agreed to train Ursula under the direction of Dr Willi Mayer-Gross, at that time Director of Clinical Research at the Crichton Royal Infirmary, in Dumfries, Scotland. Dr Mayer-Gross was formerly Professor of Psychiatry in Heidelberg. A three-year course of training was specially devised for Ursula, to include medical lectures and working with Mrs Heller, gaining experience in the wards of the infirmary. After the training period, she was appointed to the staff and worked as an assistant to Mrs Heller for four years, teaching groups of up to 25 patients who were suffering from a wide variety of mental illnesses.

She then moved to London and introductions from Dr Mayer-Gross brought her into contact with other eminent psychiatrists who referred patients to her in a practice which they had helped her to set up in Park Street, and later in Wimpole Street. She also received referrals from Consultants in many other disciplines, including gynaecology, rheumatology and general medicine. In time, Ursula began teaching classes of patients, nurses, physiotherapists and lay people in many parts of the British Isles.

The training that Ursula had undertaken with Gertrude Heller had been academically taxing and practical, but because there was no official school, and she had been Gertrude Heller's only student, she could not offer any form of validated, documented proof of attainment to prospective employers. The NHS establishment did not recognize her skills, and therefore, could not employ her, but because patients were referred to her by Consultants, the BUPA private medical insurance scheme agreed to pay her fees.

Ursula wanted to use her skills in a wider setting than just private practice and she also realized the need for research into the method which she had by then been using for more than twenty years. It was through the intervention of Lord Craigmyle, who had witnessed the effects of Ursula's work and realized its value, that the Albertus Magnus Trust was set up by those sympathetic to her cause. With income from the Trust, Ursula was able to undertake work as a volunteer therapist and was appointed to the Oxford Regional Pain Relief Unit, working there between 1981 and 1982.

In 1982 Ursula moved to the Sir Michael Sobell House hospice in Oxford, where a research programme was set up for her by Dr Robert Twycross. The results were published in *The Practitioner* in 1985.

Next she moved to the Royal Free Hospital in London, joining the Academic Department of Surgery in 1984, at first teaching women with breast cancer and then, increasingly, patients with other diagnoses. She was able to help many surgical patients with a wide range of symptoms and problems. A pilot study was carried out on patients suffering from intermittent claudication, examining the effectiveness of the method in helping them to give up cigarette smoking; the results were very encouraging. With the certain knowledge that cigarette smoking is the main cause of intermittent claudication and its potential aftermath of lower limb amputation, it is to be hoped someone in the future may be able to take up the programme and save many young men from this sad fate.

Her last research programme, a large study using the relaxation method for patients undergoing hysterectomy or cholecystectomy, was nearing completion when Ursula died.

During her years at the Royal Free Hospital, Ursula gave workshops and lectures at many hospitals and in many settings. She also wrote articles for medical and lay journals and books on pain control and religion. She made the audiocassette tapes 'Relax to ease pain' and 'Relax to concentrate' for patients using her technique and sometimes she would record the actual teaching sessions as they took place for specific patients, or she would record sessions for a single patient's specific needs. Copies of the original tapes made by Ursula Fleming are available by post from: Ursula Fleming Tapes, PO Box 2111, Hove, East Sussex BN3 5JX, England. For details of workshops, courses and new recordings of the lesson scripts in this book made by Carol Horrigan will be available from (please send a stamped addressed envelope): PO Box 587, Uxbridge UB10 8YE, England.

She appeared to be unstoppable, constantly working with the total commitment of someone who has implicit faith in what they are doing – giving interviews to the press, making television and radio broadcasts, taking her method to schools of nursing and physiotherapy, and to hospices and monasteries. Her total dedication to her cause was recognized in the award of the prestigious UK Templeton Prize for her extraordinary contribution to the comfort of the sick and dying. She was chosen by a team of judges headed by the Duke of Edinburgh. And yet, throughout this time she had also married, raised four successful children and had known the pain and sadness of the death of her husband.

Early in 1992 planning for Ursula's school was far advanced and she was trying desperately to continue with her work, putting her technique through the ultimate personal testing. During the previous five years she had undergone surgery and radiotherapy for both uterine and then breast cancer. Eventually she developed a rare form of leukaemia. Her nurses assessed her pain to be intolerable because of the bone involvement from the cumulative effects of her disease, but Ursula was able to control the pain and showed few outward signs of distress. She died on 17 March 1992.

Ursula once said in an interview that she believed her thirty years' work thus far was only a beginning, and that the method was so strong it would prove itself to be effective. This book, too, is only a beginning. You will find within it explicit instructions on how to learn this simplest of all relaxation methods, but more than that you will find guidance and insight into a philosophy of caring, one which helped Ursula Fleming continue to strive for the comfort and peace of patients even against the ridicule and hostility so often aimed at pioneers and those who would challenge long-held beliefs.

Fear is essentially looking ahead with dread, and the dread is of pain, the pain of sorrow or loss, or of physical suffering.
Living with any sort of fear is not living – it is partly living.

Ursula Fleming, *Grasping the Nettle*

Why the Fleming Method?

Introduction compiled from the writings of Ursula Fleming

The method can be used in many different situations

The Fleming Method of relaxation is not, like many other methods, restricted to static contemplation. It is also concerned with spontaneity of movement, developing powers of concentration, learning to reduce pain and suffering, learning objectivity in seeing and hearing, learning to control self-consciousness and learning responsiveness in interpersonal relationships.

It is safe, and can even be used by people who are mentally ill provided that, like any other patient, they can understand the instructions for the technique. This is possible because this method makes sure that the student does not lose contact with immediate reality. Indeed, the aim is to bring the student into contact with the present moment and to discourage fantasy and the dissipation of distracting images and ideas.

The method can be used in almost any situation. It can be taught to small children who are ill or frightened, to actors suffering from first night nerves, to people taking their driving test, even to women having difficulties with conception because they are inhibited by anxiety.

It has been used in hospices and in hospitals to help terminally ill patients to cope with their pain, to help people come off drugs and give up smoking, to help nurses take blood from patients after repeated efforts to do so had failed, and to help surgical patients cope with postoperative pain and distress.

The achievement of effortless concentration

The method can be used to improve efficiency in every field of human endeavour because it teaches improved concentration – concentration without tension. Tension inhibits performance. The achievement of relaxed and effortless concentration is of enormous value in everyday life.

In using the word concentration I do not use it in reference to an external active discipline where one part of the mind is under the direction of another, but as a description of *the absorption of the whole mind*. This state can only be achieved where there is no emotional conflict. If we are conscious of an emotion which is not a direct reaction to an external stimulus, but is generated by our own thought patterns, we are commenting on an experience which has already passed. We are looking backwards, and as a consequence we look forward either with relish or with fear to a repetition of it. Our concern is not with time in the present but with time past or time future. If we are wholly concentrated on our experience in the present, no part of our mind is free to make predictions or value-judgements. The most obvious example of this state is during orgasm; it is only after the event that we can reflect upon it. But the times when we are wholly absorbed in the reality of the present moment are rare. For the most part we live in a twilight world concerned either with prediction or retrospection.

Concentration is something that can be learned, a discipline in which we can be trained. It is comparatively easy to bring the body into a state of quiescence but it is much more difficult to control the mind. Thoughts automatically pass through the mind in quick succession and any attempt to suppress such thoughts and random images by force is nothing but an attempt by one part of the mind to control another part. This results in conflict, which generates tension. Energy is wasted and concentration is lost. The solution is to replace these superficial, aimless thoughts by an immediate and natural awareness of reality.

For the person trying to achieve concentration nothing must be taken for granted, so that even the confidence felt when lying on the floor that the floor will uphold the weight of the body becomes an immediate experience based not on theoretical knowledge of the law of gravity or on previous empirical evidence but on direct awareness. Letting the weight go down to the floor and relaxing any tension that impedes this process leads to the discovery that it is in fact safe to do so.

Thought is a comment on reality. When the teacher asks the students to turn their attention to the present moment they are not being asked to *think* about it but to *experience* it. When they have learned to rid their minds of random images and fruitless anxieties (as they can learn to do with this method) their concentration becomes focused and they are able to reach an open awareness of the present moment to which they can now react spontaneously. They have become capable of experiencing objective reality.

Experiencing objective reality and learning to accept what cannot be avoided or altered

Anyone who is bored or frightened or depressed tends not only to see each day as a dreary repetition of what has happened before, endlessly grey and predictable, but also to fear what the future may bring. The Fleming method enables the student to let go of each moment as it goes by and to accept each new moment in all its objective reality, no matter what it may bring. This is learning how to travel through and with time without fear.

This does not mean neglecting to plan for the future but simply accepting that no one can control it. There is no point in trying to cling to a cherished blueprint for the future and refusing to accept any alternative. Life has to be accepted as it is, not as how we might want it to be. A revolution must come about in the thinking of the student. Of course, where change for the better is possible we may do everything we can to bring it about. But where circumstances are intractable, instead of trying to escape the reality of the situation, or lamenting the unavoidable misfortune, the positive reaction is to relax, accept the inevitable and deal with it.

According to the Oxford dictionary 'to accept' means 'being content to receive', and it is exactly in this sense that the word is used here. Contentment implies an attitude without emotional opposition or conflict. The physical symptom of conflict is tension.

Eliminating unnecessary tension

Tension is not all negative, and relaxation is not in opposition to it as the good is to the bad. We have to tense muscles in order to move and breathe. I do not undervalue this sort of tension. The tension which is damaging is that which is caused by doubt and fear. If there should be a bull charging at you across a field it would be perfectly natural to react with a high degree of tension. Adrenalin would be released into your bloodstream and you would run as fast as possible. But in society today people are too often in a state of residual tension of which they are unaware, which is communicated to others (unwittingly), and which is caused by a nagging anxiety that a bull, or its equivalent, *might* appear.

Before learning to eliminate this unnecessary tension the student must develop an acute sensory perception in order to become aware of it. From adolescence onwards most of us find our use of our bodies becomes increasingly mechanical. As long as it functions adequately and without causing us pain, we tend to take it for granted.

Learning to slow down the over-activity of the body and the automatic thinking of the mind is a process of development which begins with the recognition of how much energy is dissipated in the attempt to build up protection against imaginary dangers.

If medically and physically possible, the training starts with the student lying on the floor, though the method is easily adaptable. It is of the essence of this technique, however, that the student should eventually acquire the ability to achieve a state of calm receptivity at any time and in any place or situation, quite without further help from the teacher.

When the students first lie down on the floor they often wriggle and squirm in an attempt to find a comfortable position. They may complain that the floor is too hard, but by the end of the first session several of them may apologize for the fact that they fell asleep during the lesson! They may be reminded of their complaints of severe discomfort in the first few minutes. The hardness of the floor has not altered one iota during the time that they have been lying on it. The circumstances have not changed but the students' reaction to these circumstances has become very different by the end of the session.

Here is the key to the control of pain. If, like the hardness of the floor, the cause of pain that is felt cannot be removed, the only way to deal with it is to change the subjective reaction to it. The success of the students in changing their reaction to the hardness of the floor is shown by their ability to lie quite comfortably on it by the end of the session. This gives the hope for the future that they will be able to change and control their usual tensing reaction to the discomfort, pain, distress and grief that we all experience during our lives.

Learning to control pain

Perhaps the most important application of the therapy is that it can be used to teach the patient how to control pain – not only physical, but also mental and emotional pain. The first requirement is to relax physically and to accept rather than to run away from the pain. Then comes the realization that pain and fear go hand in hand. Fear is always looking to the future in the expectation of pain. Fear generates fear and the physical signs of it are manifested in the body. The sequence spirals inexorably, and this must be reversed.

To tell a patient not to be afraid achieves nothing. The way to control fear is to control the symptoms in the body. We don't say 'I think afraid', we say 'I feel afraid'. We feel it in the quivering of the breath, the gritting of the teeth, the clenching of the hands, the sweating and the shaking. This *can* be controlled by relaxing the hands, the jaw, the breathing, and letting the weight of the body go down with gravity, then focusing the attention on the sensations experienced in the present moment, not wasting time and energy imagining what might happen in the next moment or the next day, but holding concentration on each moment of time as it occurs, on each new breath, listening to it, feeling its effects throughout the body. This is what is real. What is going to happen in the future, in the next moment, or the next week, will only be real when it does happen. Until then it can only be fantasy, a product of the mind as it dwells on its fears. Focusing attention on each moment as it occurs makes it possible to achieve a state of relaxation even in extreme circumstances.

Once the hands, the feet, the head and the breathing are more relaxed, patients should be asked to focus attention on the area where they feel the pain, noticing how they isolate it, keeping it still, protecting it, preventing the movement of breathing from going too near to it. They must learn to reverse this, breathing through the pain and into it, thus spreading the sensation through the whole body, concentrating also on those parts of the body which are not in pain. Each sensation is taken as it comes and fear of what it might become is dispelled. With each breath the patient learns to let go more completely, getting rid of the tensions generated by fear, and allowing the body's own defence against pain (the endorphines), to go about their work unimpeded.

Visualization and other distractions have their place, but they are able to reduce pain only temporarily. Controlling the breathing, relaxing and concentrating on the sensations in the body as they appear can remove the anticipation of pain. By letting go of the fear of pain many of those who learn this technique can relax in their everyday activities confident that they will be able to control and to live with their discomfort or pain.

Becoming independent of the teacher

The method requires practice, although some relief may be experienced from the first lesson. Each step in the training is working towards the students' gaining greater certainty about the method and its application in different situations. Once learned, the method can be used in any situation in which tension causes problems, from the pain of a fracture to the taking of an exam. Those who persevere with the training will find that they are using the method unconsciously every hour of the day and that it can change their attitude to life, improve their efficiency in dealing with life, and alter for the better their relationships with all around them.

The role of the teacher is only temporary. Proof of the efficacy of the training comes with personal experience, and it is the ambition of the teacher to reach a stage at which the student will say, 'I don't need you any more.'

Notes for teachers

Observations by Ursula Fleming

Preconceived ideas about the method

Some students already have a fixed idea about what I purport to teach before they come to me, and often it is very difficult for them to give up this idea. Their minds are closed, and they learn nothing new. Acceptance means that whatever happens you accept it and you learn through it. It is not necessarily by being good at something that you learn the most. The people who find this most difficult are often those who can relax physically quite easily, so they don't know what they have to change – they still have to grasp what is missing. A certain amount of humility or at least a certain open-mindedness is required not only in the student but also in the teacher.

Being relaxed as a teacher

The essence of teaching is not the transference of information from one brain to another; it lies rather in the teacher's ability to assess the feedback (often unspoken) of his or her students and to react to it. The teacher who is only concerned about presentation, cannot react spontaneously to the situation, and consequently, his or her teaching will be very superficial.

When I am teaching, I never use a script. I prepare *myself*. I make sure that I am relaxed, that I am sufficiently free of my own self-awareness to be able to direct my attention to the needs of those I am teaching and react to them spontaneously. I have no preconceived ideas about the direction in which I want a session to proceed. If I did, then I would have little contact with the reality of what is happening. If I am prepared, I am relaxed and concentrating. I enter the room full of people and it doesn't worry me at all. I am neither concerned nor interested in the impression they have of me. It is only what I am teaching that has importance – not me.

Tension and self-consciousness

Every thought generates some emotional energy which is expressed, however subtly, by our body language. If there is tension in the room, the best means of calming a tense situation is to remain calm; the words that you use are comparatively unimportant.

I allow each session to proceed as it will. I prepare myself for each encounter. If I think that a group or individual may be less than cooperative then I spend some time before embarking on the session coming back into reality so that I am not anticipating what may happen and therefore communicating my anxiety to the students. By anticipating, I would lose the ability to concentrate on their reactions for I would be too engrossed in my own. In this way, the students are observing the method in action although they are, at this point, unaware of the teacher's inbuilt concentration and control.

When the students become still and close their eyes they are virtually alone, but the fact that no one is looking at them except the teacher takes some time for them to realize. They tend to imagine the way they look and fear that they may appear foolish. The word 'self-conscious' is sufficiently accurate. They are preoccupied with the image they think they must be presenting. The students' reactions are apparent to the teacher from the visual signs – a slightly nervous smile, a general air of tension, the awkward way that they position their bodies, as though they were composed of separate autonomous parts which had been clumsily joined together. Gradually, as their attention is drawn to these bodily symptoms of unease, they become less concerned with visualizing their appearance from the outside; they become focused and are concentrating.

Concentration and its loss

What has surprised me on several occasions has been the observation that one person losing concentration has transmitted this slight agitation to other members of the group who were so situated that they could not have been aware of this in any auditory or visual sense. A group of students lying on the floor gradually become totally concentrated. The difference between this state and going to sleep is, at first, difficult to distinguish, but after a time, the students learn how to calm the associative automatic-thinking and filtering areas of the brain and how to turn their attention to the coordination of mind and body. This gradual development is visually apparent to the teacher or any acute observer. The faces smooth out, the bodies relax and a stillness comes over the room which is almost tangible. But, if one student should open his or her eyes, even making no sound, and look around, before long, the concentration of the whole group will be broken. I offer no suggestions which would explain the mechanics of this means of communication but I have seen it happen so often that I feel it is no coincidence.

The challenging or frightened student or patient

Occasionally there will be one member of a group who is obstructive, challenging the method by questioning in detail or making aggressive remarks. After a time the other students may become annoyed by this and their concentration will be affected. I treat such a person just the same as all the others, answering questions as they arise, and bringing the individual into the discussion. Usually this dispels the tension and the obstructiveness disappears. Some students start the sessions with the challenge that they will try it 'just this once'. Others claim that they cannot possibly lie on the floor (and in some cases this is obviously true). Others present a quiet, composed, unfathomable and distant role. In all cases I remain calm and react kindly to them all.

Sometimes patients find the very idea of relaxation threatening and they may refuse to continue with it. My teacher had a patient who had not walked for many years and spent all of his waking hours in a wheelchair. After a time, and following intensive relaxation sessions with her, he found that he could move unaided, but it frightened him so much that he refused to continue with the sessions. This is an extreme example of how we can be unwilling to change ourselves: we would rather live in a known misery than cast ourselves out into the unknown. This is why I believe that the essential quality for learning the method is courage. Letting go of our protective tensions can be very threatening, because of the thought of the frightening possibilities of what may happen when they are lost. Asking students to do this is asking a lot, but they must consider the alternatives. Either they can continue to run away from their situation and bury themselves in a fog of drugs and fear or they can tackle it head on and do something about it. Learning the method can be tiring and uncomfortable at first, but everyone can choose their own pace and I believe that 'gently' should be the watchword – each person should be enabled to let go in their own time. Gradually it becomes apparent that each of us can let go a little more than we did before, without being eaten by up guilt and with control over our fears.

Closing the session safely

At the end of a session always ask the patient or the group members to stretch slowly, turn on to their side, and sit up before they slowly stand up in their own time. Although there is no altered sense of consciousness in the method, and it leaves the participants feeling alert and not drowsy, they may still have a slight drop in their blood pressure. In order that no one experiences feeling faint there should always be enough time left at the end of the session for everyone to move at their own pace. Time should also be given for feedback and discussion of any problems, observations and comparisons.

Reactions to learning the method: my own experience

I found lying on the floor threatening in the extreme when I first started learning relaxation. I had no conception of what was real and preferred to experiment with any fantasy rather than accept the conventional idea of reality, which I would discount with logic anyway.

I stopped lying down. My teacher was kind but firm, which was what I needed. I knew that it was cowardly of me, and when I lay down again, I was in a much easier frame of mind and found it more bearable. I wanted to question everything, even the reality of the floor, but our own existence cannot be proved intellectually. At first, every attempt at sensing even the contact of my body with the floor was supremely difficult, because I questioned whether I really felt it or not (everyone does this). Also, I visualized all the time, so that I was very rarely concentrating fully. On the occasions when my brain at last became subordinated to my senses, the relief was enormous and I found it a very secure experience. I then stopped thinking that relaxation was in some way amusing and my teacher rather ludicrous. I became totally convinced of its usefulness.

I had been prescribed a strong drug to induce sleep and I found that I was now able to stop taking it without much hardship. I found that my moods lifted, but I did experience episodes of anxiety and panic. Gradually I tracked the cause of these down to my mind and body connections. Fear of my fear was causing more fear and it was all a vicious circle. I could feel fear as an immediate disturbance of my breathing, it was never relaxed. Always, I visualized it and counted its rhythm as one would count bars of music.

Although I was told repeatedly to make less effort, I still thought of relaxation as something to be achieved. Eventually I felt I was getting the message, but it was happening in phases. I suddenly realized how simple it is to have relaxed breathing, simply by not putting up any opposition to it. Then I would bring to mind a cause of being frightened and I would feel enormously better. I had learned to control my panic by relaxing and becoming more extroverted. I always found that my eyes were the last to relax, but when they were, I could always see things much more independently of my own jaundiced view of life. If I was feeling low, everything looked grey. When I relaxed my eyes this changed and gradually my mood would lift too. I came to realize that it is possible to control emotions by relaxing the body.

Introduction to the lessons

The following lessons are based on transcripts of sessions given by Ursula Fleming when teaching nurses and other people who were *well and physically fit*. They would then practise the method themselves before teaching it to others.

It is important that Lessons 1 and 2 are taught first as they are pivotal to all that follow. Once the basic technique is mastered the remaining lessons can be added to a student's repertoire in any sequence according their suitability to that individual's needs and abilities. In an ideal situation anyone learning the technique would benefit most from experiencing the whole sequence of lessons, however, some of the more physically challenging lessons can be omitted for students who are already in pain. Many nurses suffer from chronic back pain and would need to take the lessons in a sequence in which they feel comfortable. They will still be able to use the technique with as much effect. Patients with breathing difficulties may need to use Lessons 1 and 2 with adaptations and then follow on with Lesson 7, which specifically addresses the use and control of breathing.

Some lessons include lying on a broomstick to elicit the experience of pain and mild discomfort for those students who are not in pain or who have never experienced severe pain. This may seem extraordinary, and indeed it is quite unique to the Fleming Method, but there is no doubt that it is a very safe but powerful experiential technique for differentiating between pain, discomfort and sensation. Obviously, there would be no need to include this exercise in any programme devised for a patient who already has severe pain, but it can be used for patients who may be expected to experience increasing pain or discomfort as their disease or therapy protocol progresses. Alternatives such as using pressure on the arm can be devised for individual patients whose disabilities prevent them from lying on the floor.

The scripts for the series of lessons have all been retested and amended for comprehension, where necessary, using thirty-five volunteer patients at The Middlesex Hospital in London, and accounts of some of their experiences with the method are given in the final section of the book. The class experiences and exercises have been carried out by twenty groups of nurses in both pre-and post-registration education. Many of the patients and nurses had used other relaxation techniques. Without exception, they found the Fleming Method easy to use and helpful, and those who had used other techniques, such as meditative or tense–release methods as found in Jacobson (1938) found it easier to learn and more effective in use. Between them, the patients and nurses covered the range of problems that can be helped by using the method as described by Ursula Fleming in her notes.

To begin with the scripts should be read as far as possible as they are printed, although minor adjustments for dialect and cultural differences can be made by the teacher using them. Time should be allowed to elapse between the phrases as indicated by five dots thus ..... About 4–5 seconds is usual, but this can only be a guideline. The pause allows the student to hear and process the information or instruction and the teacher must use discretion in judging how individuals are reacting within any session. When longer pauses are needed in the more advanced lessons suggested amounts of time are given in the instructions.

The scripts should be delivered in a clear and gentle tone, but it must not be hypnotic (Bernstein and Borkovec, 1973). The students should not become soporific in the lessons as they will miss some instructions and will not benefit from the session. Keeping a focus on the content of the session should keep participants awake (Lichstein, 1988; Kokoszka, 1992), although some would argue that any patient who falls asleep during a session must need to rest (Fanning, 1988). Conversely, if you are teaching a group of twenty or more in a large room and you have the type of voice that becomes shrill when raised, it is suggested that you use a good quality microphone and address system, tested before each session to ensure that no 'feedback' noise interferes with the relaxation. If you are unfamiliar with sound systems, ask for assistance from a competent technician in the field.

A therapeutic environment will enable both student therapists and patients to benefit more from learning the technique. The teaching room should be warm but well ventilated, because relaxation cannot be achieved if participants are tensing their muscles against the cold. Have good lighting, but, if possible, not bright fluorescent lights overhead. The floor ideally should be carpeted, but if it is a smooth surface it must always be clean. People cannot relax if they are aware that their clothes are becoming soiled. For the purist teacher and student, Ursula Fleming's method can be applied verbatim, that is, without any softening of the hard floor. Sometimes, however, a compromise must be made (see also Ursula's case histories in the final section). Several of the nurses who took part in the retesting of the method were extremely tired and could not tolerate the pressure on their tense scalp from the hard floor. Rather than have them abandon the sessions or discard the method after the first day, I allowed them to use gymnasium mats or a small thin cushion for their head, but only initially, and only for those people with a great deal of tension in their scalp. As students become familiar with the method and proficient, they can dispense with these aids. I also adapted the method for those of my patients who were already very ill or unable to leave their bed or wheelchair (Levin, 1987; McCaffery, 1983; Sims, 1987).

Working with people who have health problems

Developing a long-term or life-threatening disease with myriad symptoms to contend with can bring a sense of frustration that most people can only imagine. Helping someone to cope by developing their control mechanisms has been identified as a care priority (Kelly, 1984; Mooney, 1991; Murphy, 1983). Symptom control is a high priority for all patients: they want to make their disease just part of their life. By teaching them techniques which will enable them to participate actively in their care, it is hoped that they will begin to experience a better qualify of life despite their illness (Deatrick, 1990; Walding, 1991; Walston, 1991). Giving patients the freedom to choose how they will participate in their symptom control is their right, and part of the health care practitioner's role is to aspire to attain as high a quality of life as possible for each patient in his or her care (Varrichio, 1990). Indeed, Padilla and Grant (1985) found that patients related quality of life to whether it was worth living and that it is a measurable outcome of care.

When introduced to a patient as part of a total lifestyle package, learning to use the technique before expected symptoms appear will enable the patient to be in control as soon as they do, and Ost (1987), in a review of eighteen controlled studies, found that being able to use relaxation as a part of everyday life in many different situations confers long-term benefits. For the patient, this could mean using fewer drugs, which often have unwanted or unpleasant side-effects, whilst controlling the main symptoms (Houldin et al., 1991). Even when strong analgesic drugs have been accurately titrated they may still affect levels of awareness and consciousness, and therefore render the patient less able to communicate with visitors when they arrive, depriving them not only of a sense of control, but of the vital need to interact on a social level.

Beginning with a simple relaxation response where there is no altered state other than a heightened sense of awareness, the lessons rapidly allow the student to develop a sense of control, and in doing so, they demonstrate clearly to the user the interdependence and interaction of mind and body. The confidence to control unpleasant symptoms and sensations rapidly expands as students become aware of the empowerment they have gained at very little expense of time or effort (Beck, 1976), and by using simple relaxation, a method which can be more effective than hypnosis in altering physiological parameters (Paul, 1969).

Health care practitioners are ideally suited to teaching the Fleming method because they are aware of the stressors that beset their patients on a daily basis. They should be able to integrate their detailed knowledge of the anatomy, physiology and pathophysiology of their patients' disease processes with their understanding of the psychosocial factors affecting the individual needs of the patient. As can often happen, for reasons beyond their control, nurses may have to work within a remit for which they have not received specialized training. For example, a patient with learning difficulties may be admitted for surgery, or a pregnant woman admitted to a medical ward for stabilization of endocrine problems. In these cases, advice must be sought from the relevant specialist before beginning the sessions regarding approach and any special precautions that must be observed. Usually there will be few if any problems, but all health care practitioners are accountable to their professional bodies for standards and quality of care and have a duty to their patients in implementing that care at the highest level of proficiency. All practitioners who wish to add the Fleming Method to their armoury of caring techniques and support mechanisms are also advised to study and practise the method personally and with willing non-patient volunteers (colleagues, relatives and friends), until they have become thoroughly conversant with the programme, the dialogues and their effects. Using relaxation techniques to help patients to control symptoms is not regarded as an extended role and only requires a professionally trained person with adequate skill and experience in the technique to implement it as part of patient care (Karle and Boyse, 1985; Lichstein, 1988). Such a practitioner is described by Holmes (1991), who believes that interaction of this kind embodies qualities that can influence the implementation of a new concept. The practitioner would be able to persuade patients to participate in a new method of self-help, implement the educational requirements of the approach and thus help patients attain their recovery goals. These were the aspirations of Ursula Fleming when she helped her patients to learn and use her method.

In a study carried out by Schain (1980), it was found that patients want to work *with* health care professionals to regain their health and maintain their independence, rather than simply being passive recipients of care and therapy. Therefore caution is also advised regarding the efficacy of the method and the potential for over-enthusiasm. It must be recognized that although it is a powerful tool in symptom control, it is not a panacea, and should never be indicated as a cure in any way. Such a course of action would only be detrimental to the reputation of the practitioner, and subsequently to the method itself (Lichstein, 1988).

Finally, practitioners must be aware of the emotional effects and outcomes of any relaxation technique in both the patient and the therapist.

Deep feelings can be released (Hough, 1991), with anger sometimes directed at the relaxation therapist (Abrowitz and Weizeberg, 1978), or anxiety increased (Bernstein and Borkovec, 1973; Heide and Borkovec, 1984). Support for the practitioner from a colleague, group or qualified therapist is recommended, but especially if the practitioner finds he or she is being affected personally by the patients' responses. This may not be evident at first, and many nurses especially believe that they should not and do not require the help of a counsellor or other support mechanism (Lichstein, 1988; Smith, 1992). Ursula Fleming herself talks about this factor in her reflective notes, and how she would have liked guidance at times from other members of the health care team (see Case History section).

The ever-growing literature on the relationship between mind and body is an encouraging sign that the caring professions are re-focusing on the patient as a whole and not on the separated physical and psychological entities of the Cartesian philosophy adopted and perpetrated for so long by the medical fraternities (Frank, 1985; Geden, 1989; Hillhouse and Adler, 1991; Holden-Lund, 1988; Houldin et al., 1991). The latest studies in psychoneuroimmunology are producing fascinating results which offer a scientific basis for the long held beliefs in bi-directional, mind–body interaction and interdependence, and thus support the concept of holistic care (Hamilton Birney, 1991; Van Nguyen, 1991). The implementation of the Fleming Method of relaxation and concentration can also demonstrate the powerful effects that the mind can exert upon the body, and vice versa.

> Clench your fists very tightly. Notice how other parts of your body tighten up in sympathy. After a time you will feel the first stirrings of anger. What has happened is that your body has adopted one of the sensory patterns of anger and the emotion has been generated . . .
>
> I do not believe that anyone can quarrel while their hands are relaxed . . .
>
> Ursula Fleming, *Grasping the Nettle*

The Lessons

Each lesson comprises an Introduction from the Editor, in which the teaching material and instructions will be supported by examples from recent literature and, where possible, research. This is followed by Instructions for that lesson, complied from transcripts of tapes, notes and writings of Ursula Fleming and adapted by Carol Horrigan.

The Introductions can be presented to students in any way that the teacher prefers. They include background information, rationale and expected outcomes. The Instructions for the lesson itself can be adapted to accommodate local dialect or if the teacher feels uncomfortable with individual phrases. Ursula Fleming stressed the need for spontaneity and sensitivity to different audiences, never using a 'script' herself, but therapists not yet fully experienced in the method should for the most part read and use the lessons as they are.

The scripts are printed using five dots to indicate that a pause should elapse between statements to allow the student to assimilate the instruction, complete the movement and experience its effects. Five seconds minimum is suggested as a guideline, but therapists must react to the needs and responses of individual patients and groups. Intervals of 10 seconds minimum are indicated by five dashes, and longer intervals are specified where appropriate.

Teachers should look at the advice regarding working with groups with specific needs and working with children on p. 97 before practising the technique with any students.

Lesson 1

Relaxation lying down I

> I don't want you to be just visibly immobile but to still everything in the mind and body which is engaged in useless activity.
>
> Ursula Fleming

Introduction

This lesson introduces the basic relaxation technique which underpins the whole course. It can be used alone as a method of stress control and will be used before each of the other sessions in a condensed or varied format, to initiate and remind the students of the feeling of relaxation. The main focus of the lesson is on the student trusting their own feelings and body sensations (Peper and Williams, 1981) so that they can differentiate between tension and relaxation in various parts of their body (Mitchell, 1987). Students are given time to develop their perception of their physical and emotional reactions to stress and to concentrate on the present, releasing them from the fears and anxieties which are the basis of tensions. Becoming self-aware through observation of body and mind interactions demonstrates to the students how they can actively cope with stress, not simply avoid it (Bond, 1986; Burnard, 1992; Stevens, 1971; Tschudin, 1991). By carrying out the exercises they will be able to make their own observations of the physiological functions that can be altered by thought (Snyder, 1985). In the course of the lesson, instructions are given to move the arms and legs. These movements are made to elicit awareness of tension and the positions of the limbs, and are not tense–release movements as used by Jacobson and many other workers in relaxation where the student causes each muscle group to contract and relax in turn as part of the training routine (Jacobson, 1938, 1964, 1970). They do not, however, use the contraction to cause a relative state of relaxation following tension as described by Bernstein and Borkovec (1973), wherein a 'pendulum' effect is created – the stronger the contraction of the tensing muscle, the stronger would be the relaxation which followed, thus 'producing' a relaxation response (Lehrer *et al.*, 1988). Relying on the body's ability to recall sensation, position and tensions in everyday movements, the Fleming Method is supported by recent research carred out by Lucic *et al.* (1991), who found that actually tensing muscles was detrimental to relaxation.

Instructions to students

First, take off or loosen anything which will prevent you from relaxing, for example shoes, belt, watch, glasses, rings and bracelets.

Find a space and lie down on the floor . . . . . make yourself comfortable.

During the exercises that I am going to ask you to do, I just want you to experience your body's responses and sensations . . . . .

Don't analyse them or have any preconceived ideas about what to expect. I will not ask you to do anything difficult or dangerous. Just listen to what I say and try to carry out each step as I say it . . . . .

Place your trust in your own ability to carry out an instruction, to experience your own reactions and to analyse them later . . . . .

If you try to analyse them as you go through the sequence, you will lose the continuity and flow of the exercises . . . . .

Close your eyes . . . .

Turn your attention to your body . . . . .

Not 'looking' for anything specific or expecting any strange sensation . . . . .

Accept what it is like, simply lying as you are . . . . .

Let it slow down . . . . . slowly . . . . . very slowly . . . . .

There is no need for any activity . . . . . except breathing . . . . .

Observe your breathing . . . . . don't change it . . . . .

When you think about it, you will always change it . . . . .

But for the moment . . . . . just let it flow . . . . .

Accept it as it changes to my suggestion and then let it go back to its normal rhythm . . . . .

Feel the weight of your body . . . . .

When we hear the word 'weight', we tend to visualize the word first, then what it means to each one of us . . . . .

Don't think about what your own weight means to you in any way except the gravity that is holding you down on the floor . . . . .

Think about what weight *is* . . . . .

Weight is caused by the pull of gravity . . . . .

Don't resist the pull of gravity . . . . .

If you resist it, you will create tension . . . . .

Let your weight go to the pull of gravity . . . . .

Let your weight go onto the floor . . . . . feel as if it is going *into* the floor . . . . .

Allow your body to become as heavy as possible, giving in to gravity . . . . .

Each time you breathe out, let gravity make your body a little more heavy . . . . .

Feel the weight of your head and neck . . . . .

Your head is just another part of your body . . . . .

It *is* the control centre for your body, but just for now, think of it as no more important than any other part of your body . . . . .

Just for now, let your body work on its own . . . . . without any instructions from your head . . . . .

Think of your head as simply a case for your brain, and your face as a flat surface made of skin and bones . . . . .

You do not need to show expressions at the moment . . . . .

Allow your face to rest . . . . .

Allow your eyes to rest . . . . .

Don't visualize anything . . . . .

Look into the darkness inside your head and accept this . . . . .

Withdraw inside yourself . . . . .

Don't concern yourself with anything outside your own skin . . . . .

It is as though you are alone . . . . .

Don't watch yourself . . . . . don't think about what you may look like . . . . .

Don't even wonder if you are relaxed . . . . .

Become completely absorbed in the sensations that you can feel
. . . . .

Have no value-judgements about whether they are good or bad   .
. . . .

Just accept them . . . . .

Don't expect anything . . . . .

Let your body be . . . . .

Just let it be . . . . . *(pause for 5–10 seconds)*

Before you can do anything about learning to control your body,
you must get to know it better . . . . .

You must become literally more sensitive to it . . . . .

Develop a greater sense of perception . . . . .

Not just when there is something seriously wrong, but noticing
subtle changes in muscle tension and breathing patterns during the
day . . . . .

To begin learning this control, first concentrate on your right
arm . . . . .

Turn all your attention to it . . . . . don't visualize it . . . . . or move
it . . . . .   .

Feel it . . . . .

Feel its weight . . . . .

Its warmth . . . . . even your pulse

Feel the contact with the floor . . . . .

Lift your right forearm on to your elbow . . . . .

Notice how your mind immediately cuts in . . . . .

Wondering if you are doing it the same as everyone else . . . . .

Whether you are doing it 'correctly' or making a fool of yourself   .
. . . .

Your concentration has been interrupted . . . . . you are no longer
alone . . . . .

You are now concerned with the effect you are creating . . . . .

Of what others may be thinking of you . . . . . your movements are mechanical . . . . .

Let the arm fall . . . . . don't lower it gently or push it, just let it fall . . . . .

Notice whether you made a decision to control the movement or predict the outcome . . . . .

Or did you simply give in to gravity and let it fall? _ _ _ _ _

No harm will come to you, and yet you are tempted to control the falling. We are so conditioned to self-protection that even when we know there is no danger, we still cannot completely 'let go' . . . . .

Try the movement again, but before you lift the arm, notice how, in preparation for the movement, energy flows into your arm and hand . . . . .

Let it happen . . . . .

Let the arm become so energized that it almost lifts itself . . . . .

Notice too how you breathe in as you lift the arm and breathe out as you let it fall . . . . .

Compare the sensations in your right arm to those in the left . . . . .

Whether you are more aware of those in one arm or the other . . . . .

Now do the same movement with the left arm . . . . .

Lifting the forearm on to the elbow . . . . . and letting it fall . . . . .

Compare the sensations in it to the right arm . . . . .

And once more with the left arm . . . . . lift it on to the elbow . . . . .

Be aware of the sensations . . . . . and let it fall . . . . .

Compare both arms once more . . . . .

Don't have any ambition . . . . . there's no 'right' or 'wrong' way to do it . . . . .

You feel what *you* feel . . . . .

Being in the moment with your body . . . . .

Aware of *your* sensations - - - - -

In this technique you are making yourself open to new experiences
. . . . .

If you have preconceived ideas . . . . . then you will not learn anything
new about *your* body . . . . . *your* responses . . . . .

Accept everything you feel . . . . . good or bad . . . . .

Once you accept everything as it occurs, any strain will go . . . . .

Tensions will be released . . . . . because nothing is expected of you
. . . . .

Not even by yourself . . . . .

Often we find that it is easier to learn something if it is difficult
. . . . .

In the arm exercise you wanted to let it fall, but if you found it
difficult, you have to investigate what it is that inhibits you . . . . .

This is an example of how our minds work in conjunction with our
bodies both encouraging and yet inhibiting them, and how it is
possible to alter the process by observation, relaxation and trust.

Next, draw your right knee up, keeping the sole of your foot on
the floor . . . . .

Don't visualize anything . . . . .

Notice how the position of your body is slightly altered . . . . . your
back is more in contact with the floor . . . . . and your shoulders are
pressed down . . . . .

Let your foot slide very gently away from your body, so that
your leg is returned to its original position and your foot is relaxed
and slightly turned out . . . . .

Check that you are not visualizing . . . . .

That you are not outside of yourself watching what you are doing
. . . . .

It is important that you are *feeling* the position and the sensations
in your leg . . . . .

Compare it with the sensations and position of the left leg . . . . .

Notice whether it feels different . . . . . and how . . . . .

Notice how much more aware you are of the right leg than the left
. . . . .

That it is more relaxed . . . . . rests more easily . . . . .

That it even feels longer than the left leg! . . . . .

   It is the discovery of yourself and the way things work in *you*
that is important . . . . .

Not the way you look to anyone else outside . . . . .

What this may involve in the future . . . . . or anything else . . . . .

   Come back to the present moment . . . . .

So that you have neither anticipation of the future nor thoughts
about the past . . . . .

You are only concerned with what is happening *now* . . . . .

   Keeping the right leg completely still . . . . . it needs no energy
now . . . . .

Draw your left knee up, keeping the sole of the foot on the floor
. . . . .

Notice again how your body moves and contacts the floor as you
do this . . . . .

Stay in this position and experience how your body *feels* . . . . .

   Let your foot slide away from your body . . . . . bringing the leg
back to its original position . . . . .

   Keep your attention centred on the reality of the sensations that
you are feeling in each moment . . . . .

Don't think about the future . . . . . or the past . . . . .

Use only the energy that you need for breathing and the movement
that you are doing . . . . . at this moment . . . . .

   Don't visualize unnecessarily . . . . .

Notice only if your attention is broken when you have finished the
movement . . . . .

And come back to the moment . . . . .

Back to the gentle rhythm of your breathing . . . . .

All the time let go . . . . .

Let go more than you thought possible . . . . .

More than you may think decent . . . . .

You may need courage for this . . . . . all your inclination is to hold tight . . . . .

To hang on to something . . . . . to hang on to the tension . . . . .

We maintain a state of tension so that we can be prepared for any unspecified danger . . . . . but there are no dangers here . . . . .

You don't need to hold on to the tension . . . . .

Have the courage to let go . . . . .

Surrender all your weight to the floor . . . . .

Become still . . . . .

The only movement in your body that you are aware of is the movement of your breathing . . . . .

Don't anticipate the future . . . . . not even for a second . . . . .

Don't even anticipate your next breath . . . . .

Because every breath you take is different . . . . . unique . . . . .

Don't think about it . . . . . let it happen . . . . . let it flow . . . . .

Just feel each breath as it happens . . . . . in the moment . . . . .

Don't try to influence it in any way . . . . . accept the variations as you breathe . . . . .

In every breath you take . . . . .

Just for a few minutes remain in the stillness . . . . .

Smooth out your brow . . . . .

Let your eyes rest . . . . .

Relax your jaw . . . . .

Have the courage to let go . . . . .

That is all you need . . . . .

The courage to accept the reality of the present . . . . .

Without any fear of the future or the past . . . . .

Being still . . . . .

Being in this moment . . . . .

Use this technique whenever you feel stressed, agitated or fearful. If possible remove yourself from the source of your stress, and if you wish, you can go to sleep. You will wake refreshed and relaxed.

Before opening your eyes, stretch out as much as you can . . . . . turn on to your side . . . . . wait a few moments . . . . . and sit up before standing up.

The Dali Lama once said that we should be grateful for our enemies, because it is through them that we are given the opportunity to learn. If you think of your enemies as fear, anticipation or stress, it will be because of them that you are learning this technique. Once you have mastered it, you can then apply it to any other stressful or painful situation which could become another enemy.

Lesson 2
Relaxation lying down II

How am I to control my mind?...Thoughts come from nowhere – my body may be in England but my thoughts in Tibet.
The answer comes as I centre myself. My mind gradually slows down simultaneously with my body as I 'come to my senses'...
Gradually I come back into the present. Whatever I may be thinking about it is unreal. It is a comment on experience and I am concerned only with the experience itself.

Ursula Fleming, *The Desert and the Marketplace*

Introduction

One of the most important aspects of using this relaxation technique is learning to track any tension as it happens in the body. This is sometimes referred to as 'scanning for tension' (Everly and Rosenfeld, 1981; Charlesworth and Nathan, 1984; Kermani, 1990; Lucic, 1991). One cannot have a calm body and a tense mind – it is not possible. Once tracked, tension can be released or re-routed through the body and used as energy. The exercises in this lesson are used to create just such an effect.

There are many relaxation and meditation techniques which seek to find a sense of calm by asking the subject to think about visualizations – cool water, beautiful countryside, and so on (Cobb, 1984; Carty, 1990; Donovan, 1980; Vines, 1988). Such techniques encourage fantasy and some people find them useful as an escape from reality. Initially they are easy to use, and patients who begin to learn a visualization technique while their symptoms are few or mild will be able to use it effectively. Although based in the fantasizing that all children indulge in during times of stress, these techniques have often been discouraged or disregarded, being criticized as 'childish' or time-wasting. At the stage when symptoms are already troublesome visualization requires a great deal of imaginative input and effort by the patient and often the benefits cannot be sustained. The person is then again alone with their stressor, their escape route no longer working for them. Therefore these methods are of limited value, especially for the patient in pain or with long-term symptoms to control. Calmness can only be found inside and it does not depend upon images that only serve to cover up the real problem.

The real problem is fear, and fear is only conjured up by visions of what might happen, based on real experiences or imagined situations. Beck (1984) describes this potential for anxiety/depression as being caused by 'wrong thinking', and both Ellis (1962) and Beck (1984) attribute it to self-blame or irrational responses to past or future events. Getting rid of the anxiety which is a symptom of fear releases tension and brings a feeling of freedom. When muscle tension in the body is controlled, and stressful images are not allowed to proliferate in the mind, a true state of relaxation can be achieved. By this method a cognitive and emotional direction mechanism is activated, which Benson (1976) found to be as effective or superior to rest in his study of the relaxation response to meditation. Stress management by this method of 'feeling' for body position, tension and thought control (Beck, 1984, Ellis, 1962; Kelly, 1955; Lichstein, 1988, Strongman, 1987) can be achieved by the Fleming Method, and has been described by Meichenbaum and Cameron (1983) as 'self-talk'.

The Fleming Method is simple to learn and use because instead of starting the relaxation by trying to control the mind, the student is helped to relax the body – the mind will then want to follow.

Meditative techniques all work in the opposite direction, with the mind being stilled by the use of a monotonous sound or mantra, relaxing the body as a consequence. Some meditation teachers and practitioners believe that the word or sound used has relaxation significance, but others, including Benson (1976), argue that it is the passive attitude to the method used and not the sound itself which is significant.

Ursula Fleming repeats many times in her lessons the words 'let go', encouraging a relaxed approach to stressful situations. She admonishes her students to let go of tension, let go of tension-inducing thoughts, both from the past and future, and let themselves just 'be' in the moment of time that they are experiencing. This is not a mantra but a reminder, one which can be invoked as a trigger every time one becomes aware of tension of any kind.

If you find that your hands are often tensed into fists or you are gripping things tightly when you talk to people, this will be because your thoughts are also tense. The body always mirrors the thoughts. When patients have pain or other distressing symptoms their days are often filled with thoughts about their discomfort and its meaning, and gradually their body also becomes more tense in response to their thoughts (Kolcaba and Kolcaba, 1991). It is possible to reverse the sequence of events, however: both the thoughts and the body can be controlled into a relaxed and harmonized state.

It takes practice, but gradually students become more sensitive to the unwanted sensations and feelings in their body, change them and remain in control. To learn about the tension in the body even when lying down, students need to cultivate a sense of stillness: this means not just being visibly immobile, but being able to still everything in the mind and body which is engaged in useless activity. Many practitioners in the field have written about the importance of practice and the increased value of easier induction of relaxation in direct proportion to the amount of practice carried out (Borkovec and Sides, 1979; Hillenberg and Collins, 1983; Jacobson, 1938). Many patients find practising easy when they have a therapist with them and may not maintain their practice when they return home (Borkovec and Sides, 1979). Both Ursula Fleming and the Editor have found this to be a problem and it can be partially overcome by giving patients either tape recordings of their own sessions (provided they were made under quiet conditions and do not have background noises on them) or pre-recorded tapes of the method, although these can become irritating and soporific if used too often. The patient is far better served by being encouraged to practise to a realistic diary, which will bring satisfaction and skill enhancement.

Instructions to students

First take off or loosen anything which will prevent you from relaxing.

Lie down on the floor . . . . . make yourself comfortable and close your eyes . . . . .

Observe your breathing and let it flow . . . . . feeling a sense of energy as you breathe in . . . . .

And relaxing as you breathe out . . . . .

Do not resist the pull of gravity . . . . .

Allow your body to be pulled down by gravity . . . . .

Letting your whole weight go on to the floor . . . . .

Let your eyes rest . . . . .

Looking into the darkness . . . . .

This is what is real . . . . .

Any images which appear in your mind are not real . . . . .

They are just images . . . . .

You cannot see when your eyes are closed . . . . .

Images are a product of your imagination . . . . .

Let them fade away . . . . .

Come back to the reality of the darkness . . . . .

Images are just a comment on reality . . . . .

They are concerned with the future or the past . . . . . not with the now . . . . .

Let your mind rest in the darkness . . . . .

Let your mind rest . . . . . and let your body . . . . . be still . . . . .

You can't force your mind to be still, if you try you may become even more tense . . . . .

You can't force your mind to be still . . . . . but you *can* teach your body to be still . . . . .

Once your body is really still with your head relaxed . . . . . then your mind will be stilled . . . . .

Slowly lift your head about an inch from the floor . . . . .

Gently rest it down again . . . . .

Let go of the idea that your head is the most important part of your body . . . . . it's nothing special . . . . . just another part of your body . . . . .

Feel its weight . . . . .

Go into the darkness inside it . . . . .

And withdraw all the energy swirling about inside . . . . .

Let it rest . . . . .

Release the tension in your neck . . . . . and allow the energy in your head to flow down into your body . . . . . and spread out gently into your limbs . . . . .

Every time you breathe out . . . . . feel the whole weight of your body and head surrender to the pull of gravity . . . . .

Release the tension . . . . .

Let go . . . . .

This is what is real . . . . .

Feel the gravity . . . . .

Don't analyse it . . . . .

Just feel it . . . . .

Pulling your weight down to the floor . . . . .

Feel it and be grateful for the pull and the earth beneath your body . . . . .

Don't try to pull away from it . . . . .

Let your whole body relax . . . . .

Let your whole weight go as you breathe out . . . . .

Let your body *be* . . . . .

Just let go of the tension and let your body *be* _ _ _ _ _ _ _ _ _ _

Breathe out as deeply as you can and don't breathe in again for a few moments . . . . .

Relax in the stillness in between . . . . .

Keep calm as you breathe in . . . . .

There's no hurry . . . . .

Your next breath in will automatically happen if you hold on to the out breath for too long . . . . .

Usually we don't breathe deeply enough . . . . . we are in too much of a hurry and take short breaths in . . . . .

If you breathe out as far as possible and relax . . . . .

The next breath in will be completely automatic . . . . . and deeper . . . . .

Breathe from the abdomen . . . . . not the chest . . . . .

Your abdomen should move as you breathe . . . . . not your chest or shoulders . . . . .

Look into the darkness . . . . . and notice how your senses have become more acute . . . . .

Let your breathing happen automatically . . . . .

Feel the hardness of the floor . . . . .

Feel the weight of your body . . . . .

As you breathe out let your whole weight go on to the floor . . . . .

Keep your attention on your body . . . . .

Breathe in and feel the air filling your lungs . . . . .

Bringing oxygen which helps your body make energy . . . . .

As you breathe in, imagine that energy filling your right arm . . . . .

Lift your right forearm slowly on to your elbow . . . . . and let it rest . . . . .

Let it fall to the floor . . . . . the hand and wrist totally relaxed . . . . .

Compare the two arms – does the right arm feel different?

Don't visualize it . . . . . just *feel* it . . . . .

Each time you do this it will feel different . . . . . let it happen . . . . .

The quality of the movement and how it feels should not be from any preconceived idea . . . . .

Follow each breath and accept what happens . . . . . don't reject anything that you feel . . . . .

Lift the right arm on to the elbow again and rest it . . . . . now let it fall . . . . .

Compare how it feels with the left arm . . . . .

Turn your attention to your left arm . . . . . and repeat the movement,

As you breathe in, feel the energy move into the arm . . . . .

Lift it on to the elbow . . . . . and as you breathe out, let it fall . . . . .

Compare it with the right arm, which has had two movements . . . . .

Repeat the left arm lift once more . . . . . and let it fall . . . . .

Compare the two arms again . . . . .

Bring your attention down your body and into your right leg . . . . .

Feel its weight and warmth . . . . .

As you breathe in, slowly bring the knee up . . . . . keeping the sole of the foot on the floor . . . . . until your knee is upright . . . . .

Take your attention to your back and spine and feel the difference in position . . . . .

Breathe out and allow the leg to slide back down and the foot to roll outwards . . . . .

If you find your mind wandering and filling with thoughts of the past or the future . . . . . you will find tension creeping into your muscles . . . . .

Come back to the reality of your body and what you are feeling *now* . . . . .

Surrender to that reality . . . . . don't let fantasy take over your thoughts . . . . .

Come back to the floor beneath you . . . . . the air around you . . . . . the constant steady movement of your breathing . . . . .

All this is happening *now* . . . . . in this moment . . . . .

Reality is not locking yourself inside your body and letting your mind wander . . . . .

Reality is each moment in time . . . . .

Each breath of air you take . . . . .

Each sensation as you feel it and accept it . . . . .

Whether it is good or bad . . . . . accept it . . . . .

If the floor seems hard . . . . . accept it . . . . .

Don't just endure it because that means you are waiting for it to end . . . . .

Acceptance means letting go . . . . . making no distinction between the way it is and the way you would like it to be . . . . .

All the time letting go . . . . .

As you breathe in . . . . . draw your left leg up . . . . . keeping the sole of the foot flat on the floor . . . . .

Feel how you move your back and head to do this . . . . .

As you breathe out . . . . . let the leg slide down and the foot roll out . . . . .

Compare how the two legs feel now . . . . .

Don't think of these movements as a form of gymnastics to be counted . . . . .

Each time you do them they will be different . . . . .

Each time they will give you feedback on how relaxed you are at that moment . . . . .

And you will learn something new about your own tension every time you do them . . . . .

Notice how movement is an extension of stillness . . . . .

Don't think about it . . . . . have no preconceptions . . . . . let it happen . . . . .

If you have preconceptions about how it will be or how it should be, then you will not learn anything new . . . . . you will only confirm what you already know . . . . .

Lie still . . . . .

Let every muscle in your body relax . . . . .

Don't think about what I've been saying any more . . . . .

That has already gone . . . . .

Come back to the present . . . . .

To what is happening now . . . . .

Listen to your breathing . . . . .

Look into the darkness . . . . . don't visualize . . . . . look into the darkness . . . . .

Feel the difference in breathing in and breathing out . . . . .

Breathing in is the influx of energy . . . . .

Breathing out is letting go . . . . .

Letting the force of gravity draw you to the earth . . . . .

And between breathing in and breathing out . . . . . there is a well of stillness . . . . .

A deep quiet within you . . . . .

It spreads around your body every time you breathe in . . . . . and out . . . . .

It is always there for you to draw on . . . . .

Feel that stillness . . . . .

Follow it every time it is released into your body . . . . .

Return to the centre of your body . . . . .

To the well of stillness . . . . .

In the quiet of your centre . . . . .

The real centre of peace and control in your body . . . . .

Not in your head . . . . .

Withdraw from your head . . . . .

Withdraw from your brain and its ceaseless thoughts . . . . .

Find the stillness within you . . . . . every time you breathe out . . . . .

And rest there . . . . .

   You don't have to try . . . . .

All you need to do is let go . . . . . *(allow 10–15 seconds for the students to experience the sensation they have created)*

   Before you open your eyes, stretch out as much as you can . . . . . turn on to your side . . . . . wait a few moments . . . . . and sit up before standing up.

[Editor's note: This lesson has proved to be a most profound experience for everyone with whom I have tested the Fleming Method. It created a sense of awe in its power to relax without making the person feel sleepy or lost in time or space. Each participant said how clear and alert their thoughts were and how refreshed their body felt after completing it only once.]

Lesson 3
Lying on a stick I: the relationship between pain and fear

> If someone said to you 'Don't be afraid', when you were scared stiff, you would know, perhaps, intellectually, that it was foolish to be afraid, that it wasn't accomplishing anything, but you couldn't, by will-power alone, cease to be afraid. Whereas you can cease to be afraid if you learn to control the physical manifestations of fear. You can get over fear itself, which is a big claim to make, but try it and you'll find that it works.
>
> Ursula Fleming

Lying on a broomstick is a way of inducing a pain experience which is safe for the healthy student. *People with spinal deformity or damage should not do this exercise. This lesson would be omitted for patients already experiencing pain.*

NB: This technique must be used with caution. Pain serves a useful purpose as a warning of injury and the ability to control reactions to pain can lead to potentially dangerous misapprehension if the patient is not exhibiting any visible signs of pain. Patients who learn to control their pain with this method should always tell nursing or medical staff of any changes in the *character* of their pain, so that any necessary investigations can be carried out to prevent obstructive or neurological damage occurring.

Introduction

Pain can become obsessive. Even a small pain can begin to absorb the whole attention of the person experiencing it (Snyder, 1985). The rest of the body gradually becomes tense, totally involved with the one area of pain, and the individual cannot function. By learning to relax and accept pain as a sensation, gradually the remainder of the body – which is not experiencing the pain – will become the focus of attention instead, and the pain will be diminished in importance.

Anxiety causes tension in the muscles so that any pain perception becomes part of a spiral of anticipated discomfort, actual discomfort and finally intractable pain as the muscles increase their tension. Recognition of the initial sensation, which may be interpreted as the beginning of a pain, is the first step in controlling the ensuing stages. Once the sequence of events is interrupted, it is possible to maintain a state of relaxation in which any gradual, or sudden increase in pain perception can be changed to perception of sensations by relaxing the tension. It is recognition even of a distressing thought – which can cause tension – which can be so significant in the relaxation response. Distressing thoughts can be interrupted and any subsequent tension and pain averted by the technique.

Anticipation and anxiety about pain do not protect us from the pain any more than tensing the back muscles when attempting to lie on the stick for the first time. It can only make it worse. Lessons 3 and 4 demonstrate to the student how they can control any unwelcome sensations by means of relaxation and concentration.

The signs and symptoms of fear may show themselves in various parts of the body, but breathing is always affected. Imagining a frightening situation is sufficient to cause tension and changes in the breathing cycle. Before an interview or stage performance, people are often advised to 'take a deep breath' in an attempt to release some of this tension. If breathing is calm and controlled, then the feeling of fear is also controlled. This state cannot be achieved automatically, but can be learned and then implemented when needed.

Calming the physical symptoms of fear goes hand in hand with the understanding that fear produces symptoms that inhibit efficiency and so contribute further to the feared effect. In extreme situations, fear will gather momentum so that fear itself becomes the cause of fearful effects. A tightrope walker who anticipates falling would do so because he is not concentrating on walking the rope, but is creating fear of the future.

Learning to control fear is both a mental and physical process. Mentally, it is the recognition that fear of the future is only fantasy, and not reality which can actually harm. The situation which is feared in fantasy may never happen, and tension caused by the anticipation is a waste of energy and emotion. Reality is in the present moment of time and in the technique; the student is called up simply to deal with the situation in the moment of time that they are experiencing. Combined with control of the physical manifestations of tension, such as shallow, rapid breathing, gritting the teeth and clenching the hands, the student will master each situation and control it (Goldfreid, 1971).

Intellectually we are aware that to be afraid of certain situations is irrational, and yet there are times when the reason for fear is quite obvious. Will-power alone cannot prevent or override such fear unless the physical manifestations of the fear response are first controlled. By using this relaxation technique, the physical and ultimately the mental attributes of fear will be brought under the control of the individual. Being empowered in such a way, when traditionally people have always expected to be overwhelmed by symptoms, or at the best to have them controlled by drugs, gives the user of the technique the greatest sense of freedom (Holmes and Dickerson, 1987; Kelly, 1984; Mooney, 1991).

If the students are in fear of the pain caused by lying on the stick, then the intensity of the pain increases and they cannot wait to relieve it. By relaxing and teaching their body to accept whatever sensations are caused by lying on the stick, the pain soon 'goes away'. Lying on the stick is painful at first because the stick is straight and the spine is curved, gravity causes the weight of the body to push the curves of the spine against the stick as the body is pulled to the floor. At the end of the exercise students are asked to lie on the floor, and in comparison to lying on the stick, it will feel very comfortable. The floor will be as hard as before, but the students will have learned to relax the tension in their back muscles. They will be breathing more easily, and they will be experiencing only sensations, not pain.

Instructions to students

Each student will need to be supplied with a broomstick for this exercise.

This exercise will not damage a healthy individual; it is intended to demonstrate the difference between pain and the fear of pain. It will be uncomfortable at first until you are able to relax fully. Notice the way you react to the exercise mentally and physically.

First, take off or loosen anything which may prevent you from relaxing.

Take a stick, find a space, and put the stick on the floor beside you . . . . .

Lie down on the floor and make yourself comfortable . . . . .

Go through the basic relaxation as you did for Lessons 1 and 2 . . . . .

Attend to your breathing . . . . . bringing energy into the body on the in breath . . . . .

Relaxing into gravity on the out breath . . . . .

Don't lift them, but relax your limbs one by one . . . . .

Relax your face . . . . .

Relax your eyes . . . . .

Relax your throat and lower jaw . . . . .

Bring your thoughts back to your breathing . . . . .

Focus on this moment . . . . .

Focus on each moment as it happens . . . . .

Bring your attention to the comfortable parts of your body . . . . .

Focus on the centre of stillness within you . . . . .

Focus on your breathing . . . . .

Letting all tension go . . . . .

Being still . . . . . and at peace . . . . .

In this moment . . . . .

In your own time and maintaining your centre of stillness, push the stick under your back and lie on it so that it is under your head and your spine.

Relax . . . . . accept the sensations that you feel . . . . .

If you resist and become tense . . . . . the sensations will become pain . . . . .

Don't expect anything . . . . . have no preconceived ideas . . . . . let your body *be* . . . . .

As you breathe in, feel your body filling with energy . . . . .

As you breathe out feel it relax . . . . . relax on to the floor . . . . .

Ignore the stick . . . . .

Don't anticipate that it will be painful . . . . .

If you anticipate it, then it will be so . . . . .

If you don't anticipate pain, but you anticipate a sensation . . . . .

Then it will be just that . . . . . a sensation . . . . .

The word 'pain' is an emotive word . . . . . as soon as it is mentioned, we react by becoming tense in anticipation of a need to protect ourselves . . . . .

In order to control pain, you need to reverse this automatic reaction . . . . . to react by letting go . . . . . not tensing anything . . . . .

So do not think of the word 'pain' . . . . . pain is something which is warning you of danger . . . . .

Lying on a stick isn't dangerous . . . . .

Think of the word 'sensation' . . . . . an experience . . . . .

Our own responses to pain or pleasure are very individual . . . . .

They are the opposite ends of a spectrum . . . . .

But they are subjective experiences . . . . .

They are not reality . . . . .

They are enhanced or diminished by our expectations . . . . .

Our threshold of pain or pleasure is dependent on the degree of tolerance we adopt . . . . . – on our emotional attitude . . . . .

By adopting an attitude of acceptance there will be no emotional conflict . . . . .

Conflict which causes tension and resistance to the sensation . . . . .

Accept the situation and let go . . . . .

You will find that you become more comfortable . . . . .

Don't cross your legs or feet . . . . .

As you relax, your thighs will almost touch the floor . . . . .

Let your weight go . . . . . give in to gravity . . . . .

Ignore the stick . . . . .

Accept the sensations as they happen . . . . .

Do not anticipate . . . . . anything . . . . .

Think of it as an experience . . . . . an unclassified experience . . . . .

Observe your body if it becomes tense . . . . .

If you focus on the uncomfortable areas you will begin to think of endurance . . . . .

So don't predict sensations . . . . .

Accept what you feel . . . . . good or bad . . . . .

Do not generate self-protective tension . . . . .

Go back to your breathing . . . . .

Notice if it is easy or interrupted . . . . .

Whether your lungs feel free or constricted . . . . .

Whether you are letting the full weight of your body go down on to the floor . . . . .

Or whether you are holding it back unnecessarily . . . . .

Take your attention to your hands and arms . . . . .

Their heaviness as they rest on the floor . . . . . they are not painful . . . . .

Come back to your breathing . . . . .

To the centre of stillness inside you . . . . .

Become aware of the areas of your body that are completely comfortable _ _ _ _ _ _ _ _ _ _

Gently take the stick and push it away from you . . . . .

Enjoy the sensation of lying on the floor . . . . . *(allow a 10–15 second pause)*

Before you open your eyes, stretch out as much as you can . . . . . turn on to your side . . . . . Wait a few moments . . . . . and sit up before standing up.

Lesson 4
Lying on a stick II: acceptance of sensations and pain

> Anxiety about pain doesn't protect you from pain any more than tensing up on the stick does. It only makes it worse. Anxiety only increases suffering and it certainly doesn't ward off trouble. If anything it attracts it . . . The emotion of fear produces symptoms which inhibit efficiency and so contributes to the feared effect.
>
> Ursula Fleming

People with spinal deformity or damage should not do this exercise. This lesson would be omitted for patients already experiencing pain.

NB: Please read the caution given in Lesson 3 on p. 35.

Introduction

This lesson continues the theme of differentiation between pain and sensations and how we can teach the body to interpret pain as sensation only.

Acceptance of a sensation without pre-judging it or interpreting it as pain empowers anyone who is experiencing any of the sensations that we commonly call pains. In this lesson the student is asked to experience lying on a stick twice, but is reminded once again of the initial relaxation prior to using the stick. It demonstrates the importance of being fully relaxed and the difference it can make in controlling otherwise painful situations which may arise not only in disease, but from daily tensions (McGuigan, 1984).

Perceptions of pain are influenced by actual physiological factors such as inflammation or neurological damage but are exacerbated by the emotional needs of the individual experiencing them and the social pressures to which they are subjected (Fisher, 1988; Hearn, 1977).

Instructions to students

Each student will need to be supplied with a broomstick as for Lesson 3.

First, take off or loosen anything which may prevent you from relaxing.

Take a broomstick, find a space, lie down with your broomstick at your side and make yourself comfortable.

Begin to relax your body as you have already learned . . . . .

Keep your eyes closed, and let go . . . . .

Let both your mind and your body become still . . . . .

Feeling the sensations of weight and warmth and safety . . . . .

As you breathe in, lift your right forearm . . . . . breathe out and let it fall . . . . .

Breathe in and lift your left forearm . . . . . breathe out and let it fall . . . . .

Breathe in and draw your right knee up . . . . . breathe out and slide it gently back down to the floor again . . . . . let the foot roll out . . . . .

Breathe in and draw your left knee up . . . . . breathe out and slide it gently back down to the floor again . . . . . let the foot roll out . . . . .

Lie still . . . . . feeling each breath as it brings energy into your body . . . . .

Relaxing on each out breath . . . . .

Not looking into the future or the past . . . . .

Concentrating on each moment . . . . .

Coming back to your centre of stillness . . . . .

Keeping your breathing steady, and remaining relaxed, roll on to your side, push the stick behind you and gently roll back on to it . . . . .

Relax . . . . . don't endure it . . . . . accept the sensations that you feel . . . . .

Don't tense and wait for any discomfort to end . . . . .

Accept the sensation . . . . .

Breathe in and fill your body with energy . . . . .

Breathe out and relax . . . . .

Bring your attention to all the parts of your body that *are* comfortable
. . . . .

Discover the difference between accepting and enduring . . . . .

When you accept, you don't make any judgement between good or bad, pain or pleasure . . . . . you just let go and take whatever you feel . . . . .

Let go physically . . . . . breathe out deeply . . . . .

Accept lying on the stick for what it is . . . . . a sensation . . . . .

Nothing dangerous or alarming at all . . . . .

Feel the weight of your arms resting heavily on the floor . . . . .

Let your eyes rest . . . . .

Looking into the darkness . . . . .

Just feel . . . . . don't think . . . . .

If you think, you are just commenting on reality . . . . .

Don't question if it is right . . . . .

Whether everyone else is feeling the same . . . . .

Whether it will hurt . . . . .

Just *feel* . . . . .

Roll gently off the stick . . . . . push it away and lie flat on the floor . . . . .

Lie still and accept every sensation that comes to you . . . . . good or bad . . . . .

Don't visualize . . . . .

Look into the darkness and accept each moment of time as it comes to you . . . . .

Don't burden yourself with worries about what's going to happen or what should happen . . . . . − you cannot control the future . . . . . no one can . . . . .

You can only tackle each situation as it arises . . . . .

And the more you can rid yourself of anxiety . . . . .

The more chance you have of being successful . . . . .

Keep looking into the darkness . . . . .

Think back to when you were lying on the stick . . . . .

Did your discomfort get better or worse?

If it got even *slightly* better, then you have discovered the key to controlling pain . . . . .

Think about applying it to other uncomfortable or painful situations - - - - -

It isn't just a matter of relaxing . . . ,

By relaxing and cutting out unnecessary tension in your body . . . . . you also cut out the fear in your mind . . . . .

By cutting out fear, you bring time into perspective . . . . .

By concentrating on the reality of now rather than the nebulous future . . . . .

Pain is always worsened by the *fear* of pain . . . . .

Now gently lie back on the stick again . . . . . gently . . . . .

Don't have value-judgements . . . . .

Don't think of it as pain or pleasure . . . . .

Just an unclassified sensation . . . . .

Don't even describe the sensation to yourself . . . . .

Accept it as if it were a pattern in a kaleidoscope . . . . .

All the time moving . . . . . changing . . . . . from one pattern to another . . . . .

Watch the pattern of your own sensations change . . . . .

With an interest that is part of it . . . . . yet detached from it . . . . .

Don't try to force a change . . . . . let go . . . . . give up control . . . . .

And it will change itself . . . . . the moment you classify it . . . . .

And cling on to the classification . . . . .

And call it pain . . . . .

It will be like stopping a clock and the pain will return . . . . .

So accept the kaleidoscope pattern of sensations . . . . .

Accept the reality of now _ _ _ _ _

Roll gently off the stick and enjoy lying on the floor _ _ _ _ _

Before opening your eyes, stretch out . . . . . turn on to your side . . . . . and sit up before standing up.

Lesson 5
Balancing the stick I: calm concentration and detachment

> In a way doubt is vanity. 'Am I going to live up to my expectation of myself?' This is why I think it's important always to accept the possibility of failure. Otherwise one is always trying to stave it off. Sometimes too we want to live up to standards we set ourselves which have nothing to do with reality.
>
> Ursula Fleming

Introduction

This lesson provides an example of how we try to manipulate life and other people. By developing an empathy with the stick the student can then balance it easily on the tips of the fingers. The stick will show the student whether he or she is self-conscious, because if they are, it will immediately fall. When they are able to identify tension in their body they will be able to relax. Any conflicting emotions that they feel will be manifest in tension and they will not be at peace. The student may be able to put on a good act and outwardly appear to be peaceful; only they will be able to gauge their own stress levels by how uneasy they feel.

It is not only the hand but the whole body that balances the stick. Learning to control tension all over the body saves valuable energy and centres it ready for use.

Balancing the stick means relaxing, letting go, being utterly without tension. The quality of stillness will be transferred to the stick from the student. While the students are trying to avoid failure, they will be tense. Therefore they must accept that the stick may fall while they are reducing their tension. As soon as they become less bothered about what they are doing and what they look like, then they will succeed. The moment they watch themselves doing it, the stick will fall. Encourage students to concentrate on the partnership between themselves and the stick and not on their image, and the stick will balance.

In her teaching, Ursula often used a quotation from Count Keyserling, which endorses her emphasis on calm concentration:

> The value of learning controlled quiescence cannot be doubted. All strong minds are marked by the fact that they are not fidgety, that they can relax and concentrate at will, and that they can give their concentration to one problem more continuously than weaker minds.

Instructions to students

Each student will need to be supplied with a broomstick for this exercise. Quiet instrumental music may be played during this session.

First, take off or loosen anything which may prevent you relaxing.

Find a space and lie down, with your stick nearby.

Begin to relax your body as you have already learned . . . . .

Attend to your breathing . . . . .

Relaxing on each out breath . . . . .

Without moving them, just let your limbs relax . . . . .

Relax your face . . . . .

Relax your eyes . . . . .

Relax your throat and lower jaw . . . . .

Bring your attention back to your breathing . . . . .

Focus on this moment . . . . .

On each moment as it happens . . . . .

Focus on the comfortable parts of your body . . . . .

Focus on your centre of stillness . . . . .

Focus on your breathing . . . . . and being still . . . . . in this moment
. . . . .

In your own time, and maintaining your centre of stillness, stand up, take your stick and with your palm facing upwards, balance it vertically on your fingertips. *(Pause to allow students to carry out this instruction)*

Notice the way you are reacting to what I have just said . . . . .

You have only a limited amount of energy at your disposal . . . . .

If you use up that energy in expressing tension or fear thinking about whether you are able to balance the stick, then you will not be able to do it . . . . .

Each time the stick falls, listen to what I am saying and keep trying . . . . .

Concentration is controlling the direction of energy . . . . .

Let your hand relax . . . . .

Feel the weight of the stick carried by your fingers . . . . .

Look upwards . . . . . at the top of the stick . . . . .

Now you can adjust the movement and be prepared for changes in direction . . . . .

The moment you start thinking that it is going to fall . . . . . it will do so . . . . .

If you try to force the stick to stay upright by will-power, you won't be able to balance it at all . . . . .

Have the courage to make a mistake . . . . .

To look foolish if necessary . . . . .

The more you are willing to look foolish, the less likely you are to do so . . . . .

If you are relaxed . . . . . you adjust quite easily to the circumstances you have to face because you have to concentrate . . . . .

Your energy is not dissipated by questioning and self-doubt . . . . .

Keep looking at the top of the stick . . . . .

Some people master this more quickly than others . . . . .

But everyone learns to do it after a little practice . . . . .

One thing is certain, unless you are detached, have no ambition about it . . . . .the stick will fall . . . . .

Ambition causes anxiety . . . . .

And anxiety causes tension and that tension is transmitted into the stick from your body . . . . .

Ambition means that you are thinking about the future . . . . .

And concerned about when you will be able to balance the stick . . . . .

Both take your energy and attention away from the present moment
. . . . .

Think of the stick as something separate from you . . . . .

With its own existence . . . . .

And see the relationship between you and the stick as a partnership
. . . . .

Not as dominance by one or the other . . . . .

The moment you are *afraid* of the stick it will also fall . . . . .

Calm yourself . . . . .

Calm your eyes . . . . . calm your breathing . . . . . soften your eyes
. . . . .

If you look at the stick with eyes as hard as marbles, then you will
find that you communicate that tension to the stick . . . . .

The block is lack of empathy between you and the stick . . . . .

Feel the reality of the stick . . . . .feel its weight balanced on your
fingers . . . . .

How all the time you are reacting to that weight on your fingers
. . . . .

See the stick just as it is . . . . . not as a projection of you, as a
vehicle for your ambition . . . . .

But as it is . . . . .

Notice the things that get in the way of balancing the stick . . . . .

They are all coming from your mind . . . . .

'Am I doing this as well as the others?' . . . . .

'Do I look a fool?' . . . . .

'Will anyone laugh at me?' . . . . .

These thoughts only distract from your concentration . . . . .

And the stick will fall . . . . .

Soften your eyes . . . . . you don't really care . . . . .

Give up caring about fear of failure . . . . .

Keep balancing the stick . . . . . but don't care about if it falls . . . . .

Then your whole concentration . . . . . your whole attention can be in the moment . . . . .

This moment . . . . .

Not thinking about what may happen . . . . .

Whether you will drop the stick or not . . . . .

But being with the stick in partnership . . . . .

   Feel the weight of the stick . . . . .

Have no assumptions . . . . . no pre-conceptions . . . . .

Just feel the weight of the stick . . . . .

Just relax . . . . .

Let go . . , . let go of all defensive tension . . . . .

Then you can feel the quality of stillness . . . . .

Transferring from you to the stick . . . . .

You can feel the infinite possibilities in each second of time . . . . .

As you breathe gently in . . . . . and out . . . . .

Explore the possibilities . . . . .

Instead of getting stuck in what you think must happen _ _ _ _ _ _ _ _ _

   Please put the stick down and rest.

   Students may wish to sit or lie down for a few moments before analysing their experience of the exercise, alone or in discussion.

Lesson 6
Balancing the stick II: movement and walking with the stick

> Always check that you are not visualizing, that you are not outside yourself watching what you are doing. It is your discovery of yourself and the way things work that is important, not the way you look to anyone outside, or what this may involve in the future, or anything else.
>
> Ursula Fleming

Introduction

It is not easy for students taking part in a group session to be unconcerned about the effect they have on other people, because when they first meet, they are affected by the attitudes of the others in the group. In the beginning, each student will decide which part of their own personality they will offer directly to the others, although group dynamics will nearly always reveal their true type if they are together long enough, unless they are very good at acting a part.

As a member of a new group, embarking on a learning exercise, each person will view the others as potential competitors. The jovial, the earnest and the hesitant have all experienced the sense of wanting to be the best in a new class since they first entered school as a young child. Therefore, both the students and teachers will be pleased to note how learning the technique enables them to abandon their 'roles' as they focus on reality, lose their tensions and become receptive.

In this exercise they try to balance the stick while moving round the room to music. This exercise reveals in a very few minutes most of the students' attitudes towards other people. The aggressive, the timid and the confident will all become as balanced as their stick with the support and encouragement of the teacher. They will find an inner stability which is generated by learning the appropriate use of their energy. They develop their skill in balancing relaxation and tension in safe surroundings, which can be transferred to any situation where they wish to apply it.

Some students will doubt that they will ever be able to achieve balance of the stick or their tensions. In a way, doubt is a form of vanity, thinking about whether they will live up to their own personal expectations. It is important that they appreciate the risk of initial failure in this exercise.

Sometimes we set ourselves standards that are unrealistic and then are disappointed when we fail.

The philosophy behind the entire relaxation technique is applied in this lesson, that is, not to pre-judge, not to have pre-conceived ideas, in fact not to speculate about the future at all. The student must learn that if they can simply be with the stick at the moment that it is balanced, it will remain balanced.

Learning any new technique in a group means that someone is going to succeed quickly, most group members will learn in an average time and a few will take a little longer. The important thing is for students not to be concerned about how long it takes, but what they learn about themselves in the process.

Instructions for students

Each student will need to be supplied with a broomstick for this exercise. Instrumental music can be played during this session.

First, take off or loosen anything which may prevent you from relaxing.

Find a space, lie down and make yourself comfortable - - - - -

Begin the relaxation as you have learned in the lessons so far.

(Allow at least 10 seconds for the students to complete each instruction)

Attend to your breathing - - - - -

Let your limbs relax _ _ _ _ _

Relax your face _ _ _ _ _

Relax your eyes _ _ _ _ _

Relax your throat and lower jaw _ _ _ _ _

Bring your attention back to your breathing _ _ _ _ _

Focus on this moment _ _ _ _ _

On each moment as it happens _ _ _ _ _

Focus on the comfortable parts of your body _ _ _ _ _

Focus on your centre of stillness _ _ _ _ _

Focus on your breathing _ _ _ _ _

And being still _ _ _ _ _

In this moment _ _ _ _ _

Learning to be calm in isolation is useful, but remaining calm under any circumstance means that you are integrated and whole. You are capable of feeling safe, happy and in control no matter what difficulties life brings you.

In your own time, and maintaining your centre of stillness, stand up, pick up your stick and begin to balance it on your fingertips - - - - -

Begin to move amongst each other - - - - -

Don't think about what you look like _ _ _ _ _

Watch the top of the stick _ _ _ _ _

Don't visualize yourself _ _ _ _ _

If you worry about watching yourself, the stick will fall _ _ _ _ _

Don't worry when someone approaches you _ _ _ _ _

Keep looking at the top of the stick _ _ _ _ _

Don't move backwards _ _ _ _ _

Don't look at anyone else _ _ _ _ _

Keep calm _ _ _ _ _

And keep moving _ _ _ _ _

Come back to your centre of stillness _ _ _ _ _

If you feel tense as someone approaches, let go of the tension _ _ _ _ _

Focus on this moment _ _ _ _ _

Not on what others are doing _ _ _ _ _ but on what you are feeling _ _ _ _ _

Calm _ _ _ _ _

If you are relaxed you are no threat to the others _ _ _ _ _

You will glide past each other _ _ _ _ _

If you are tense and they try to avoid you, then you are a danger to them _ _ _ _ _

Calm yourself _ _ _ _ _

Don't be afraid _ _ _ _ _

Then you can walk close to the others and your stick will stay balanced _ _ _ _ _

If you feel any tension rising, come back to your breathing _ _ _ _ _

Breathe out _ _ _ _ _ and come back to your own centre of stillness _ _ _ _ _

Please put the stick down and rest.

Students may wish to sit or lie down for a few moments before analysing their experience of the exercise, alone or in discussion.

Lesson 7
Relaxed breathing

> If your hands are tightening up all the time you can stop it. If your breathing is tense it takes practice to straighten it out but it's fairly straightforward and all it really needs is the realization that whatever goes on in your mind is mirrored in your body. You feel this when you learn to become sensitive to it. Instead of starting by trying to control your mind you start with your body and that does the trick for you.
>
> Ursula Fleming

Introduction

In the busy lives that most people in the world lead today, many are striving to find some peace. A state of peacefulness cannot be brought about by thinking or trying to think about it. The process of thinking is too analytical. By means of thought we can understand processes, and as a result, feel confident about the prediction of future possibilities. But fears of what the future holds will often prevent us from living in the moment, tensions build in anticipation of potential future discomforts, based on previous experience, and the individual is impotent to enjoy the here and now (Kolkmeier, 1988).

 It is through the movement of breathing that we recognize life and it is through the understanding of the power of breathing that we come to a 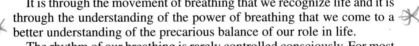 better understanding of the precarious balance of our role in life.

The rhythm of our breathing is rarely controlled consciously. For most of us, the activity of breathing can be likened to a small boat afloat on the sea: if the weather is calm, it is easy; if the weather becomes stormy, the boat is rocked and buffeted bringing sickness and fear to the occupants. By learning to stabilize breathing, it is possible to become independent of external circumstances – as a boat fitted with stabilizers is independent of the weather – and to remain at peace regardless of the storms assailing us.

Through the development of psychology as a recognized science, it has been possible to demonstrate that our emotional reactions are not always consciously controlled. The memories of traumatic experiences which we have buried in our subconscious are often the cause of conflicts which disperse our energies and dissipate purposeful activity. This is why individuals who have faith combined with a lack of doubt and who see no conflict in their actions are able to achieve great deeds and 'move mountains'. Successful people are those who are capable of focusing all their energies on a target without allowing the fear of failure to impede them.

Psychoanalysis, psychotherapy and other forms of psychological therapy have been developed with the objective of resolving these inner conflicts. By bringing conflicts to the surface, to the conscious mind, in a controlled way, and discussing them with an empathetic, trained listener, it is hoped that, eventually, the fear exacerbating the conflicts will be calmed. When this happens the results can be gratifying, but the methods all take a long time and are not effective in all cases. If they are not effective, for whatever reason, then the sufferer may be left more fragmented than before.

It is possible for patients to deceive themselves or the therapist by means of their own intricate attempts at cerebral self-analysis and non-disclosure. Although consciously they would like to be released from the anxieties and doubts that beset them, subconsciously, the last thing that they may be ready to expose are the vulnerable feelings around which they have carefully built a layer of protection for many years.

Any emotional agitation, no matter how overt or subtle, can be mirrored in a disturbance in the rhythm of breathing; the patient can deceive their mind, but not their body. When they have harnessed a true depth of calmness in breathing, then any deviation from this state can be recognized and the cause identified (Gardner and Bass, 1989; Hough, 1991; Innocenti, 1983; Salkovskis, 1988). The person can know their depth of calmness by monitoring their breathing.

Awareness of breathing in the most subtle sense can only be achieved by a technique of withdrawing from the external world and by concentrating entirely on 'following' the rhythm of breathing (Van Nguyen, 1991).

Breathing and the control of pain, panic and spasm

Either in movement or at rest, a positive flow of energy directed by breathing helps to reduce pain.

Instinctively we protect a painful area by keeping it still and tense, defending it from 'attack' by the pain. Even the movement of breathing itself is not allowed near the area of tension and the pain is isolated by tension from the ebb and flow of the energy travelling through the body as it is generated. This action intensifies pain. Protective tensions are then multiplied, spreading outwards so that even if the pain was originally in the stomach, the hands become tense, toes curl and eyes begin to lose focus in the total absorption by the pain. This form of tension serves no useful purpose; it is only exhausting – and this is true of both mental and physical pain.

Sometimes patients suffering from intractable pain suffer from muscle spasm. This may cause them to hyperventilate in their panic. They can usually be relieved of the spasm by quietly and firmly telling them to, 'Breathe out, let go, breathe out, forget about breathing in – that will take care of itself – just breathe out.'

This same method can also be used for patients in a panic over breathing difficulties, such as whooping cough, asthma or bronchitis. Combine the instructions with reassurance, also gently stroking their arms in a downward movement and, when they are a little more relaxed, stroking their forehead. The most important aspect to emphasize is the fact that the patient can do something positive to deal with the situation. Once they can remember the instructions, they will be able to implement them immediately if a similar situation occurs.

Breathing into the pain and then through it makes the pain appear to disperse throughout the body. When it is 'spread thinly' in this way, the patient can cope with it better than when it is concentrated in one area. This is especially true if the initial pain was emanating from an area of the body that the patient perceives as particularly vulnerable, such as their head or heart, or a tumour. If the patient is made aware of their total body and all its sensations, not just a small area of pain, they are able to concentrate more easily on their breathing. Once the breathing pattern is changed, they are able to become detached from the pain and think of it as a sensation instead.

Counting the number of seconds that it takes to breathe out fully is not recommended, as this can induce more panic and a sense of defeat if the patient's ability to attain certain numbers decreases if and when their disease progresses. It is far better simply to concentrate on maintaining the out-breath for as long as possible before allowing the in-breath. One technique which does have value and which Ursula Fleming sometimes used is to hum on the out-breath. As the patient concentrates on maintaining a clear, steady sound they are not concentrating on their pain, spasm or panic, and they are able to empty their lungs completely in the process.

Editor's Note: If the student finds it difficult to breathe lying down, use pillows, or they may sit in a comfortable chair with their legs supported on a footstool. People with breathing difficulties are not precluded from learning the technique, and they will feel more in control of their breathing problems once they have learned it. This is especially important for those with asthma, other long-term lung disease or severe heart disease. Do remind them, however, that a breathing technique will not cure their illness and that they must continue to use all medication as prescribed. Many people with asthma *are* able to reduce or discontinue their 'as required' drugs when they have mastered the technique and become more confident that they can cope with their lifestyle (Beck, 1984; Cox and Mackay, 1976; Ellis, 1962; Poppen, 1988).

Instructions to students

First take off or loosen anything which will prevent you from relaxing.

Make yourself comfortable lying down on the floor _ _ _ _ _

Begin to relax your body as you have already learned _ _ _ _ _

Attend to your limbs and relax them _ _ _ _ _

Allow your body to give its weight to gravity _ _ _ _ _

Let go of any tension that you can feel _ _ _ _ _

Relax your face _ _ _ _ _

Relax your throat _ _ _ _ _

Relax your eyes _ _ _ _ _

Relax your spine _ _ _ _ _

Listen to your breathing _ _ _ _ _

Knowing that each breath that you take has its own dynamic and rhythm which can be sensed in every part of the body, even in your head and feet _ _ _ _ _

It is felt not so much as a movement, but rather as an ebb and flow of energy _ _ _ _ _

When first learning this technique, pay most of your attention to breathing out _ _ _ _ _

This is usually much too shallow _ _ _ _ _

If you are anxious, you breathe in before it is necessary because the main area of tension is in your diaphragm _ _ _ _ _

It is useful to remember to breathe out - - - - -

Let the rib-cage subside as fully as possible _ _ _ _ _

And remain motionless for a few seconds before breathing in again _ _ _ _ _

When your attention is first drawn to your breathing, you become inhibited. You feel that you should breathe deeply and regularly and so you control the action in order to do so _ _ _ _ _

Don't try to control the complete breath . . . . .

Coventry University
Lanchester Library
Tel 02476 887575

Borrowed Items 30/03/2016 13:03
XXXXXX3688

Item Title	Due Date
38001002828683	20/04/2016
* Behavioral relaxation training and assessment	
38001005438027	20/04/2016
* Stretching anatomy	
38001005786177	06/04/2016
* Creative relaxation in groupwork	
38001002055642	20/04/2016
* Relaxation for concentration, stress management and pain control : using the Fleming method	
38001005048867	20/04/2016
* Relaxation techniques : a practical handbook for the health care professional	
38001005515717	20/04/2016
* Sport and exercise physiology testing guidelines : the British Association of Sport and Exercise Sciences guide	
38001005515527	20/04/2016
* Sport and exercise physiology testing guidelines : the British Association of Sport and Exercise Sciences guide	

* Indicates items borrowed today
Thankyou for using this unit
www.coventry.ac.uk

Exhale as fully as possible and allow nature to take its course
- - - - -

As long as you only do this, breathing will take care of itself
- - - - -

As the rhythm of your breathing becomes calm, your whole state of being becomes calm, undisturbed by the jagged edges of anxiety
. . . . .

When you recognize anxiety . . . . .

When the emotion of anxiety is seen to be only negative . . . . .

Then concentrate on your breathing and nothing can disrupt your serenity - - - - -

As you breathe out allow your weight to go down to the floor
- - - - -

Let go of the control - - - - -

In a moment the breath in will automatically happen - - - - -

Filling your body with energy - - - - -

It is through observing the breath that a different concept of time emerges . . . . .

Each breath is unique . . . . .

It has never happened before . . . . .

And it will never happen again in this way . . . . .

It is as unique as each moment of a lifetime - - - - -

The moment that is happening now is unique - - - - -

Not next week . . . . .

Not tomorrow . . . . .

Not even the next second . . . . . but now - - - - -

This is the only moment that is real - - - - -

Concentrating on each breath as it ebbs and flows through your body brings a sense of peace and comfort - - - - -

The movement is as basic and as essential as the movement of the waves in the sea _ _ _ _ _

Observe the energy build-up as you breathe in . . . . .

It builds to a crescendo and then overflows and withdraws back to the earth . . . . .

When breathing out is relaxed, energy is returned to the centre . . . . .

To the powerhouse of your being _ _ _ _ _

Relaxing in the stillness inside _ _ _ _ _

Lying flat and being quiet is like recharging a battery _ _ _ _ _

Energy is withdrawn from the periphery . . . . .

From your hands and arms . . . . .

From your feet and legs . . . . . eyes and forehead . . . . .

Converging on the centre . . . . .

From here, breathing in adds more energy _ _ _ _ _

And it can all be directed to wherever you need it in your body _ _ _ _ _

Breathing out allows the energy to flow toward the centre once again and as the energy is withdrawn from the hands and feet and eyes . . . . .

So too is tension drained towards the centre . . . . .

Where it can be used as energy _ _ _ _ _

The body is soft and relaxed - - - - - for you to use when you need it - - - - -

With a feeling of peace _ _ _ _ _

Any pain or tension becomes easier _ _ _ _ _

If we allow protective tensions to multiply they serve no purpose . . . . .

They are only exhausting _ _ _ _ _

Recognize them as they occur . . . . .

Feel them . . . . .

And allow them to drain to the centre and convert into useful energy
- - - - -

Each time you feel the tension return . . . . .

Breathe *out* - - - - -

Let the tension go - - - - -

Forget about breathing in - - - - -

Just let go - - - - -

And the in-breath will take care of itself when it is needed - - - - -

Let go and feel at peace in the out-breath - - - - -

Let go of tension [or panic, muscle spasm, pain, nausea, etc.] - - - - -

Let it go to the centre - - - - -

In your centre of stillness where you can control the energy as you wish - - - - -

Breathe *into* your tension [etc.] - - - - -

Allow the tension [etc.] to disperse through your body as you breathe
- - - - -

Spreading out into a thin imperceptible layer - - - - -

Until you can't feel it any more - - - - -

Before opening your eyes, stretch out as far as you can - - - - - and turn slowly on to your side and rest there for a while before sitting or standing up.

Lesson 8
Sitting in a chair: breathing and posture

> If a person sitting in the huddled position is suddenly brought good news, his joy brings about a physical response and the first thing he will do is to sit up straight.
>
> Ursula Fleming

Introduction

Before commencing this exercise the group should carry out a relaxation exercise lying on the floor as they have before each of the previous lessons. This brings their focus to relaxed muscles and breathing in the most familiar position.

When learning to relax lying down, it is easy to let go and breathe easily, but there are times when it is necessary to be relaxed alert and upright, concentrating on some activity. The need to generate energy from breathing in is then enhanced by good upright posture, with the lungs fully expanded.

Lesson 8 demonstrates how relaxed breathing can be carried out sitting in a chair and how it can relieve tension while carrying out many daily activities, such as working at a computer or answering the telephone (Jackson, 1990; McGuigan, 1984). Again, it helps relieve the breathing problems associated with asthma and other chronic lung or heart disease because it re-educates the patient's breathing habits back to using the whole of the lungs, not just the upper sections, a habit often adopted by patients with breathing problems. For example, breathing patterns may be affected when dealing with difficult situations or whilst concentrating on a task. The technique will bring an awareness of altered breathing and can be used at any time, giving the user command of their breathing under any circumstance other than an acute allergic reaction (Lichstein, 1988).

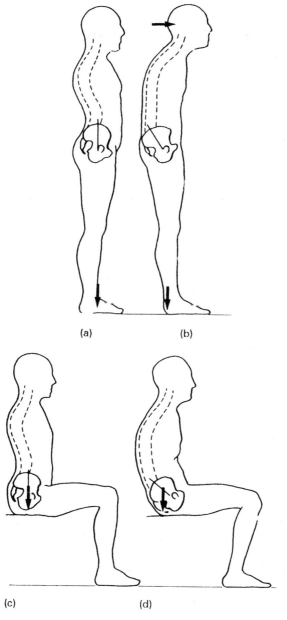

(a)   (b)

(c)   (d)

Figure 1 Correcting faulty posture: (a) and (c) show the correct position of the sacrum in standing and sitting; (b) and (d) show the incorrect position

Instructions to students

Each student will need a straight-backed chair without arms for this lesson.

This exercise begins by relaxing on the floor if possible, and is continued in a sitting position on a chair. Patients who are below average height may have difficulty relaxing if their feet do not naturally touch the floor. Give them a footstool or equivalent to keep their knees at a right angle.

NB: The students must be shown the diagram of the correct and incorrect positioning of the sacrum (Figure 1) and practise the correct posture before the lesson begins.

First, take off or loosen anything that may prevent you from relaxing . . . . .

Find a space, beside your chair, lie down on the floor and relax . . . . .

(Allow approximately 10 seconds between each instruction where indicated by five dashes)

Bring your attention to relaxing your body - - - - -

Concentrating on breathing out deeply - - - - -

And in focusing on a centre of stillness within you - - - - -

Let your eyes soften - - - - -

Your jaw relax - - - - -

Stay relaxed, concentrating on this moment - - - - -

Attend to any areas of tension in your body and deal with them - - - - -

Stay on the floor for a while - - - - -

Then in your own time . . . . . roll on to your side . . . . . sit up . . . . .

Stand up and transfer on to the chair beside you - - - - -

Sit on the chair with your feet on the floor . . . . .

Your hands resting lightly on your thighs . . . . .

Hold on to that feeling . . . . .

Don't use the back of the chair to lean on . . . . .

Think of your body as a machine that has to be working in a balanced state . . . . .

Sit upright and bring your sacrum into the correct position . . . . .

So that it is tilting forward and your spine is straight . . . . .

If you are out of balance, both your mental and physical self will be out of balance.

Close your eyes so that you can concentrate more on how this exercise *feels* _ _ _ _ _

You can't breathe properly if you are not sitting upright _ _ _ _ _

The most important area now is the lower part of your back _ _ _ _ _

The difference is between letting the sacrum sag _ _ _ _ _

Creating a backward curve in the spine _ _ _ _ _

And pulling it up _ _ _ _ _ to keep the spine straight _ _ _ _ _

Don't concern yourself with your shoulders for this postural exercise . . . . .

If you need to sit in one position for any length of time, observe your body for areas of tension . . . . .

And let them go _ _ _ _ _

Let your knees rest a little apart, so that there is no tension from trying to sit with them together . . . . .

Keep your eyes closed and sit like this for 2 minutes.

I'll tell you when the time is up.

(Allow two minutes exactly for this)

What was the most difficult part to keep still?

(Allow time for the students to respond)

It is uncomfortable, because we often don't use our back muscles, we allow chairs etc. to support us instead and the muscles become weak. However, once your muscles become accustomed to the new posture you will no longer feel pain. This will take time.

The main function to be affected by sitting well or badly is your breathing. If you are sitting badly you cannot energize your body by breathing fully, and vitality is lost.

Close your eyes again . . . . .

Whilst learning to control your posture,

Don't endure the pain but accept it _ _ _ _ _

Think of it as the opposite of pleasure . . . . . but not *pain*, just a sensation _ _ _ _ _

Breathe steadily _ _ _ _ _

And the feeling of slight panic associated with pain will go _ _ _ _ _

Panic is thinking about the future again . . . . .

Come back to the moment . . . . .

Relax into the posture . . . . .

And you can apply all the energy-moving principles of correct breathing that you learned lying on the floor _ _ _ _ _

Using the technique when you are sitting at your desk or for any other activity brings concentration as you balance between generating and using your store of energy and letting go of tension or pain.

Remember that when you are sitting, if you lean forward or back, your breathing will go out of balance again.

Re-adjust your breathing at regular intervals and gradually it will become automatic.

Allow time for questions and discussion at the end of the session.

Lesson 9
Posture and neck pain

> When the posture is upright the body is sufficiently oxygenated for the subject to be capable of positive response.
>
> Ursula Fleming

Introduction

The number of working hours lost per year owing to back and neck pain now accounts for an enormous loss of revenue in all industries in the UK and other industrialized countries. Learning to relieve and prevent the spasm and muscle fatigue caused by inappropriate use of the neck and back muscles would enable many people to resume work earlier, and prevent further temporary or permanent injury.

This lesson once again makes use of internal observation by the student of his or her own body. By teaching students to *feel* the correct positioning of the spine and neck muscles the technique enables them to make automatic minor adjustments as they become aware of faulty posture during their daily activities. After practice, they will automatically change position, and use a stretching or relaxing movement to prevent problems occurring.

Patients who suffer from chronic neck pain are often employed in jobs which necessitate an abnormal stance, or they adopt a forward-pushing movement of the chin as a postural habit.

This lesson can be taught as part of a complete set following Lessons 1 and 2 to patients who have neck or back pain. Students who have not performed the exercise in Lesson 8 should be shown the diagram of the correct and incorrect positioning of the sacrum (Figure 1, p. 65) and practise the correct posture before beginning this lesson.

Instructions to students

Each student will need a straight-backed chair without arms for this exercise.

First take off or loosen anything that may prevent you from relaxing fully.

Lie on the floor and take a few minutes to relax as you have done at the beginning of all the lessons. *(Allow 4–5 minutes for this)*

In your own time and maintaining your state of relaxation, slowly stand up, and then sit on your chair.

Sit far enough forward so that your feet are flat on the floor and your back is *not* supported by the chair. Tilt your sacrum forward. Your spine should be comfortably erect, supporting your head.

Close your eyes . . . . .

As you breathe out . . . . . let your arms become heavy . . . . .

This should be easier in this position because your arms and shoulders move fractionally as you breathe.

Make sure that your knees are relaxed . . . . .

That you're not holding them tightly together . . . . .

If you do, then tension is transferred into the abdomen from the legs . . . . .

At this stage, concentrate more on breathing *out* . . . . . breathing *in* is an automatic response . . . . .

The more relaxed you are . . . . . the less perceptible your breathing becomes . . . . .

Generally we concentrate more on the sensory input that we receive from the front of the body, and have comparatively little input from the back.

Take your attention to your spine . . . . . and feel that it is a prop that holds you erect . . . . .

Feel your head resting easily on top of your spine . . . . .

Don't push your chin up to make your head erect . . . . .

Feel instead that your spine is elongating through your neck and that it supports your head . . . . .

Don't let it fall forward like a drooping tulip . . . . .

Normally the amount of conscious bodily direction is very small in comparison to all the automatic functions which are happening whether we are awake or asleep. You are now going to change the balance just slightly in the amount of conscious control that you can have.

Try to sense your head in relation to your body . . . . .

Much of the strain which causes pains in the head comes from tension in the neck.

Gently allow your head to tilt forward as far as it will go . . . . .

Slowly lift your head back to a vertical position so that you can feel the muscles in the back of the neck taking the strain as you lift . . . . .

Hold your head steady and rest for a moment . . . . .

Now *gently* let your head go backwards as far as possible . . . . .

Probably further than you thought possible . . . . .

Then bring it *slowly* back to the vertical position . . . . .

This time taking the strain on the front of the neck . . . . .

Assess how your head feels in relation to your spine now . . . . .

Compared to how it felt before the exercise . . . . .

(The student will say that it feels more 'joined/integrated/together' etc.)

You should sense a feeling of release or relief . . . . .

You can tell whether you are doing this well by whether or not you are enjoying it. That is the only criterion.

If you are not enjoying the sensation, then there is some area of tension which is preventing it.

The same criterion can be applied to every other exercise that you learn in this discipline.

It is the way that you do the exercise that matters. If you do it mechanically, you will feel very little difference at all. But if you concentrate as fully as when you let your arm fall down to the floor in the very first exercise, not thinking about *what* you were doing but feeling every muscle stretching, if you feel your vertebrae, gradually finding the correct balance and straightening themselves out one on top of the other, you will find that the relief of the strain on your head and neck is marked.

Notice how easily your head rests on top of your spine . . . . .

It finds its own upright position, which may be very different from the one that is habitual to you.

Feel how your breathing is easier, with your head gently resting in this way . . . . .

Feel the air entering your lungs completely, without effort, and with it the energy being created by your body as the oxygen circulates in your bloodstream.

The energy being created by your body when you breathe more completely is now available for your use. At the end of the exercise you will be able to feel where this is happening most.

Keep your eyes closed . . . . .

Make sure that they are resting . . . . .

Don't visualize . . . . .

Let your eyelids be like curtains . . . . .

Blocking out any interest which is external to you . . . . .

Feel how you are supported by the chair and the floor . . . . .

Everything is still except the movement of your breathing . . . . .

Feel that as you breathe out, energy is withdrawn from your head . . . . . your eyes . . . . . even your ears . . . . .

If your body and mind are in harmony then your posture must and will be right . . . . .

Keep your eyes closed and let your hands rest on your knees . . . . . Once again, *very slowly and gently*, let your head fall forward with your chin tucked in . . . . .

Now *very, very slowly* lift it up . . . . . feeling the muscles in the back of the neck gently lifting the weight of your head . . . . .

Hold the vertical position of your head as it returns to its pivotal point . . . . .

Feel the muscles working together on opposite sides of the neck to maintain this position . . . . .

Now let your head fall gently backwards as far as you can without pain . . . . .

Allow the muscles around your neck to soften and relax . . . . . and then slowly return your head to the upright position . . . . .

Feeling the muscles in the front of your neck doing the lifting and the muscles in the back of the neck controlling the speed at which it rises . . . . .

Remember to do this several times a day . . . . .

Just looking up at the sky or a tall building for a few seconds . . . . .

Children have flexible necks and never complain of neck-ache because they have to look up at grown-ups all day long!

Return your attention to your breathing . . . . .

As you breathe in, feel the slight movement of the chest reflected in your shoulders . . . . .

and in your neck . . . . .

and in your head . . . . .

and feel it change as you breathe out . . . . .

The position of your spine is of great importance at all times. While sitting or standing, it is essential that you become aware of the difference in effect in your breathing when your spine is erect, or crooked.

When your sacrum is tilted backwards, you can feel the strain in the back of the neck . . . . . your chest also becomes tilted, and your breathing is constricted. *(This is the posture adopted by those in despair. See Figure 1.)*

To balance your spine, your sacrum must be tilted forward into its correct position. When you have corrected it, then the whole spine rests easily, the weight of your body is supported and your breathing is once more free to function as it should.

When looking for the effects of your own posture habits, feel what your body is doing in an objective way . . . . . and observe where there is stress . . . . .

Habitual faulty posture contributes to many other disorders of the spine and head, resulting in many days of lost work.

Not only does bad posture cause physical breakdown, but it can also affect your mental and emotional attitude. When your body is upright, your lungs can expand fully, your body is fully oxygenated and ready for positive responses. If you are huddled and bent over, you appear to be enduring life rather than living it to the full.

The open body is one that generates and uses energy at the optimum level. When we maltreat our bodies by bad posture, we lose this feeling of vitality and energy, a basic instinct is thwarted and we become aware of vague feelings of anxiety and frustration.

Open your eyes and stand up . . . . . feel the difference in your neck and spine.

Lesson 10

Seeing in a relaxed way

> If we see objectively our observation is much more detailed,
> and as a result our assessment of the situation in which
> we find ourselves is that much more balanced.
>
> Ursula Fleming

Introduction

Often, when we meet someone for the first time our eyes harden until we become relaxed in their presence. When we are with children or someone that we love our eyes are automatically softer (Lichstein, 1983).

We don't see objectively, we look at things not for what they are, but for what they mean to us. We look at people in the same way, asking ourselves, 'Will they harm me or will they be of benefit to me?'

We see only what we are conditioned to see: when we look at the sky, the floor, or anything – we don't see them as they are, but rather categorize them, label them and try to put them into mental bundles or pigeon-holes.

Seeing in a relaxed way is seeing without classification. After using the following exercise the students learn to see objectively, separate from themselves. With this comes acceptance and an ability to be relaxed in new situations.

Instructions to students

Each student will need a chair for this lesson.

First take off or loosen anything which may prevent you from relaxing fully.

Lie down beside your chair and make yourself comfortable . . . . .

Relax as you have for all the other lessons. *(Allow 4–5 minutes for this)*

In your own time, and maintaining your relaxed state, sit up, stand up and then sit on your chair.

The technique of really looking begins with closing your eyes . . . . .

And relaxing . . . . .

Go inside yourself, as you did before . . . . .

Into the darkness . . . . .

Shutting out the world as you normally see it . . . . .

Don't use visualization or fantasy . . . . .

This is difficult, especially if you have been trying those types of technique for relaxation . . . . .

We also automatically have visions that we like to conjure up when we close our eyes. This is a habit which is begun in childhood and we continue to use it as an escape mechanism even as adults.

Forget about vision . . . . . and go inside the darkness within you . . . . .

Relax . . . . .

Feel the weight of your eyelids covering your eyes . . . . .

Just for now don't think of yourself as you . . . . .

Think about being a functioning being . . . . .

Think about your eyes and what their function is . . . . .

Feel the energy going into them . . . . .

Feel that it isn't necessary . . . . .

And withdraw it . . . . .

You will find this easier to do if you feel the energy withdraw as you breathe out . . . . .

So, withdraw the energy from your eyes . . . . .

And take it to the centre of your body . . . . .

To your diaphragm . . . . .

Soon I will ask you to open your eyes . . . . .

When I do, feel as objective about this as if you were a camera . . . . .

I will ask you to just take the shutters away from your eyes and let the vision come to you . . . . .

We tend to see things for how they will affect us. We take vision for granted and become accustomed to what we see until we no longer see things as they are . . . . . and we lose the beauty all around us.

In a moment, when I ask you to open your eyes, do not see the vision in front of you as though it is entirely for you and how it will affect only you . . . . .

If you look at things objectively, you will see much more detail, your assessment of your situation will be more balanced. Try not to categorize what you see . . . . .

Don't tell yourself 'This is the floor, this flower is pink' . . . . . just let it come to you . . . . .

Feel how you respond to it . . . . .

Not in your head, with thoughts . . . . . but inside yourself . . . . .

Don't think 'That's a good colour' or 'What a bad colour', just be receptive to it and accept it . . . . .

Don't analyse what you think about it . . . . .

Now, *slowly* open your eyes and keep them absolutely relaxed . . . . . and soft . . . . . and see as you have never seen before _ _ _ _ _

Don't divide what you see into good or bad, be receptive to it . . . . .

Not what you might think about it . . . . .

Don't focus on one thing . . . . . don't focus at all . . . . .

Close your eyes and go back into the darkness . . . . .

Don't think about what you are doing . . . . .

Accept it . . . . .

Experience it . . . . .

When you close your eyes you are in darkness . . . . .

Experience *that* . . . . .

In a few moments when you open your eyes again, experience vision and be really absorbed in what you see . . . . .

This is concentration . . . . .

This is seeing without classification . . . . .

Practise it . . . . .

Practise it with people, when you meet them or deal with them; do not be concerned about what they think of you, whether you can trust them, or whether they may be hostile to you . . . . .

If you become concerned in this way, then you are concerned not with the other person but with yourself, Although you are seeing them, you are just watching for their reactions to you . . . . .

It is very useful to be able to see people quite objectively, separate from oneself. Not uncaring, but accepting that they are going to make their assessment of you anyway . . . . .

So let them, and then forget about it. Then you can be receptive to them instead of worrying about preconceived suspicions . . . . .

You can be totally relaxed in any new situation.

Now open your eyes and enjoy truly *seeing*.

Allow time for discussion at the end of the session.

Lesson 11
Relaxed walking

> If you feel self-conscious in walking towards us try to
> become more interested in us than in yourself. You aren't
> seeing us, you are seeing a battery of hostile eyes. We
> aren't hostile and yet you are defensive towards us.
>
> Ursula Fleming

Introduction

Most people feel self-conscious when asked to walk across a room in front of a group. Make a request for a volunteer for the first demonstration. Ask them to leave the room and return walking with the stick balanced, and then a second time without the stick. When they use the stick, their concentration will be such that self-consciousness will be diminished; when they return and look at the faces instead of the stick, they will lose concentration and their self-consciousness will be very obvious.

Real, effortless grace comes when the student finds concentration and detachment so that the walk across the room can be made without a moment's thought as to who may be watching. Gradually each member of the class will be able to take their turn as their courage builds, and they see that fellow students are actually enjoying the experience and gaining confidence (Schilling and Poppen, 1983).

Instructions to students

Each student will need to be supplied with a broomstick for this exercise. If possible, play quiet, relaxing music during the exercise. A video recorder can be used with the students' permission (see below).

First take off or loosen anything that will prevent you from relaxing.

Find a space and lie down.

Relax in your own way. *(Allow 4–5 minutes for this)*

In your own time, sit up and stand up.

Forget about being self-conscious, feel your balance . . . . .

Stand upright . . . . .

Shoulders relaxed . . . . .

Not like a guardsman with your shoulders drawn back . . . . .

But with your arms and hands loosely at your sides . . . . .

Your sacrum and therefore your lower back should be tilted forward . . . . .

This is its natural position . . . . .

Your spine is now erect . . . . .

With your head resting easily on your neck . . . . .

Feeling balanced . . . . .

Your chin is neither poking forward nor tilting backwards . . . . .

Think about the mechanics of walking . . . . .

The transfer of weight from one foot to another . . . . .

Walk around the room . . . . .

In slow motion . . . . .

Keep your knees relaxed . . . . .

Transfer your weight from one foot to the other . . . . .

Feel it roll off the back foot and how you move it forward on to the front foot.

(Allow the class a minute or two to carry out this exercise to gentle music)

Feel how minute alterations in balance through your feet help you to keep upright . . . . .

How your body is working in unison.

(Allow another minute or two for this and then ask the students to take a broomstick and find a space)

To develop the flexibility of your feet, put your stick on the floor and stand with one foot lengthways on it. Place your big toe on the stick and lay your foot along it diagonally to the heel. Relax and transfer your weight on to the stick . . . . . using your other foot on the floor just to balance . . . . .

Take all your weight on to the foot on the stick . . . . . hold the position for a few seconds and then stand on the floor . . . . .

Notice how the foot that was on the stick feels lighter and more sensitive to the floor compared with the other foot . . . . .

Change feet and stand on the stick with the other foot *(allow time for this)* . . . . . now compare feet again . . . . .

Now take your stick, and with your palm facing upward balance it on your fingertips and walk around the room again . . . . .

Concentrating on the top of the stick . . . . . but noting how relaxed your knees and feet are . . . . .

You don't need to jab your heels into the ground as you walk . . . . .

Just walk lightly over the floor . . . . .

Feel how relaxed your shoulders are . . . . .

And your hands . . . . . your jaw . . . . . your eyes . . . . .

Your whole body is moving in relaxed unison.

(Allow a few minutes for this exercise)

Please put your sticks down on the perimeter of the room and come back to the centre . . . . .

Relax your breathing and your body and simply walk about . . . . .

Feeling the difference in your whole body . . . . .

The confidence you now have in this easy movement . . . . .

The criterion for success is whether you are enjoying walking in this naturally efficient way . . . . .

Be aware of the rhythm of your breathing co-ordinating with the movements of your body . . . . .

The flexibility of your feet . . . . .

The flexibility of your legs . . . . .

And the positive sensation of moving forwards in time and space . . . . .

Relax your eyes . . . . .

Become receptive to everything around you . . . . .

Accepting everything that you see uncritically . . . . .

Not expecting anything . . . . .

Not seeing things as good or bad . . . . .

Just seeing them in this moment . . . . .

When you are walking somewhere with a purpose in future . . . . .

To the bus stop, to work, to visit someone . . . . .

Maintain this relaxed rhythm . . . . .

Try to remain relaxed, thinking only pleasant thoughts . . . . .

Accepting what you feel and see in the moment . . . . .

Do not allow your walking to become overburdened with worries and fears for the future . . . . .

As soon as you do, you will feel the tensions building again . . . . .

In a tense state, the present ceases to exist for us . . . . .

We are engulfed in care for the future and the anxieties we generate are reflected in our bodies and movements.

Ask the students to leave the room in twos or threes, and return to walk past the group, first with the stick and then without it. Talk them through the experience (see below). Having guidance as they carry out the exercise will give them not only instruction but feedback to boost their confidence. A video recording can be useful to show the students how much they have improved, but they must agree to be filmed. If they are coerced or feel obliged to do so, then their movements will reflect their reluctance and tension at all stages of the exercise and the objective will be lost.

Some groups will agree without hesitation but you will have an equal number of groups for whom a camera would be a substantial threat. In order to win their confidence, it is useful to mention the idea of video at the beginning of the course of lessons; then, when they have become more familiar with each other, they are more likely to agree willingly.

(As they leave the room)

When you are outside the room, go through your relaxation, concentrate on your breathing, using the out-breath to relax. Concentrate on the moment that you are experiencing, don't have any preconceived ideas about what will happen, don't think about the future, or what others think of you. Find your centre of stillness and return to it if you find your thoughts straying.

(As they re-enter the room)

Look at the top of the stick . . . . .

Forget about being self-conscious . . . . .

Let your eyes soften . . . . .

Don't think about the impression you're making . . . . .

Feel your breathing . . . . .

Feel your body moving across the floor . . . . .

Let your eyes take in what they see . . . . .

Try not to project anything . . . . .

Not even a nonchalant attitude . . . . .

Just be receptive to what you see and hear . . . . .

And the sensations of your body . . . . .

Any tensions that you feel are communicated to us . . . . .

Any protective act that you use will be very obvious to all of us watching you . . . . . just as a dog can sense that you are frightened of it . . . . .

Accept the fact that you feel awkward . . . . . and vulnerable   .
. . . .

Let the physical symptoms relax . . . . .

Concentrate on the sensations that you feel now . . . . .

The floor beneath your feet . . . . .

The relaxed movement of your body as you walk . . . . .

Seeing the room with its shapes and contours . . . . . the colours . . . . . the light and shade . . . . . the people in the room . . . . .

The stillness and activity in the room . . . . .

The stillness in you . . . . .

Feeling how you are in this room . . . . .

Walking through time and space . . . . .

Letting go . . . . .

Repeat the script for each group. End the lesson when all the students have completed the exercise.

Allow time for discussion.

Lesson 12
Advanced techniques for relaxation I: the body roll

> Don't think of these movements as gymnastic exercises. It isn't the quantity that matters – the number of times you do them, but the quality ... it isn't the achievement of movement which is important. It is what you learn about movement itself – and you can go on learning for the rest of your life.
>
> Ursula Fleming

Introduction

As we breathe, the physiological effect can be felt in every part of the body. Breathing in brings air into the lungs where oxygen is extracted from it to be used by all the cells of the body as part of its energy-producing mechanism. Therefore breathing in can be likened to an influx of energy and breathing out as a withdrawal into restfulness.

When the student carries out the exercises in the earlier lessons, they experience lifting each forearm and allowing it to fall. They naturally breathe in with the lift, and out with the fall. Yet, allowing any part of our body to fall is going against the protective conditioning which we develop and are trained in from infancy, and to decondition ourselves to be relaxed in falling requires concentrated attention on the direct sensory experience. In the arm exercise, the arm is held upright and in balance by the synchronized tension in the opposing muscles. The moment the decision is made to let the arm fall, this tension is released, and immediately the arm falls. The slightest premeditation or inclination to ensure the safety of the arm will result in some of the muscles retaining their tension and the arm will be 'lowered' rather than allowed to fall.

A further development of the arm-falling exercise is to allow the whole body to fall. The first stage is to practise a simple roll in which, from lying on the side, the body is allowed to fall on to the back.

Performing the exercises mechanically serves no purpose. The number of times they are performed is of no consequence, but the quality of each experience should continually improve. Allowing the body to fall, even in the body roll, takes courage, and a combined physical and mental release which comes from total trust in relinquishing all control and abandoning judgement of the future.

Instructions to students

Play quiet, gentle music throughout this lesson.

First take off or loosen anything which may prevent you from relaxing fully.

Lie on the floor and use the relaxation techniques that you have already learned. *(Allow time for this and use the following script to guide students)*

Close your eyes and relax all your limbs _ _ _ _ _

Each time you breathe out allow your body to become more relaxed _ _ _ _ _

Give your weight to gravity _ _ _ _ _

Not looking to the future _ _ _ _ _

Or back into the past _ _ _ _ _

Concentrating on this moment _ _ _ _ _

Feeling your jaw relaxing _ _ _ _ _

Your eyes softening _ _ _ _ _

Feeling calm and safe _ _ _ _ _

Returning to your own centre of stillness _ _ _ _ _

Letting go of all tension _ _ _ _ _

The only feeling of movement in your body is your breathing _ _ _ _ _

Letting go of all tension _ _ _ _ _

Just letting go _ _ _ _ _

Stretch your right arm above your head, and turn on to that side, resting your head on the outstretched arm . . . . .

Lie in that position for a few moments and relax again . . . . .

Gather your energy with a deep in breath . . . . .

Let your head fall gently backwards off your arm on to the floor . . . . .

And let your whole body roll backwards to follow it . . . . .

Lie still and breathe steadily . . . . .

Coming back to your centre of stillness . . . . .

Repeat the movement several times . . . . .

It should become a smooth, flowing movement . . . . .

Think about movement being 'rest drawn out in an orderly sequence' . . . . .

Take your time to begin and complete the movement smoothly . . . . .

Concentrate on maintaining your relaxed state . . . . . rest between each movement.

(Allow the students approximately five completed movements)

Now turn on to your left arm and lie for a few moments relaxing . . . . .

Gather your energy with a deep breath . . . . .

Let your head fall gently backwards . . . . .

And roll on to your back . . . . .

And relax . . . . .

Going into your centre of stillness . . . . .

Repeat the movement several times . . . . .

Rest between each one.

(Allow the students approximately five completed movements)

If you enjoy this exercise, then you are completely relaxed; if there is any strain, you need to practise more.

Lesson 13
Advanced techniques for relaxation II: the controlled arm lift

> The reason I started learning relaxation by this method was that I had never met before a science which actually teaches concentration. How to focus your energy. And that's what it does. You are over-tense because you are expending energy uselessly in ways that are not productive. You can learn to control that so that you have all the energy you need centred for when you need it.
>
> Ursula Fleming

Introduction

This exercise uses the slow lifting of one arm and its controlled lowering to the floor over a period of approximately 5 minutes. It enables the student to experience the fine-tuning of concentration on one single area of the body. The sensations which occur during the exercise demonstrate the difficulties that can be encountered in both simple and complex concentration situations. Students can then use the experience in any situation where close concentration is required of them. It is not a tense–relax mechanism.

Instructions to students

This exercise can be used following the body roll or as a separate exercise. Play quiet, gentle music throughout the lesson.

Take off or loosen anything which may prevent you from relaxing fully.

Find a space, lie down on the floor, with your arms by your sides, and relax in your own time. *(By now the students should be able to take themselves through the relaxation sequence automatically, using the sections of the exercises that they prefer and are able to use most effectively.)*

Continue to concentrate . . . . .

Remember that 'movement is rest drawn out in an orderly sequence' . . . . .

Lie in relaxed concentration . . . . .

Bring your attention to your right arm . . . . .

Breathe in deeply and feel the energy move into the arm . . . . .

Very *slowly* lift the whole arm from the shoulder . . . . .

When it is vertical to the floor *(allow time for all the students to complete the movement in their own time)* . . . . .

Very, very, slowly lower it back down . . . . .

Until it rests again on the floor . . . . .

Move it evenly . . . . .

Feel the strain as you lower it . . . . .

It may feel as though the floor is moving away from it as it gets closer . . . . .

When the arm is on the floor . . . . . compare the sensations that you feel in both arms and shoulders . . . . .

Be aware of the changes that took place in your whole body as you carried out the exercise . . . . .

Notice how the movement affected those changes . . . . .

How you could control the changes . . . . .

Take your attention to your left arm . . . . .

Breathe in deeply and lift the whole arm from the shoulder until it is vertical . . . . .

And *slowly* lower it back down to the floor . . . . .

Very, very slowly . . . . .

Don't let your attention wander from the arm and its sensations . . . . .

When it is finally back on the floor, compare the two arms again . . . . .

Rest and relax . . . . .

The next sequence takes 5 minutes in total, from lifting the arm to when it is at rest on the floor again.

Bring your attention again to your right arm and once more, as you breathe in, taking about 2½ minutes, keep breathing steadily and bring the arm *slowly* to the vertical - - - - -

In your own time, beginning as you breathe out, and as slowly as possible (about 2½ minutes again), bring the arm back to the floor.

(Allow 5 minutes in total for the students to complete the movement. Continue the script to maintain their attention and to encourage them as they perform the exercise)

Breathing gently and steadily as you lower the arm - - - - -

Feeling the energy being brought to the arm each time you breathe in - - - - -

And feel the air around it as you lower your arm slowly - - - - -

Keep concentrating on that one arm - - - - -

Lowering it at an even pace - - - - -

You will find it a strain at the top of the arm - - - - -

Don't speed up the pace as it becomes more strenuous - - - - -

This is an exercise in concentration - - - - -

If you complete the movement quickly it is because your concentration wavers, not because it is painful - - - - -

Concentrate on relaxing _ _ _ _ _

On breathing _ _ _ _ _

Bringing the energy to the arm _ _ _ _ _

Notice how other parts of your body are reacting to the movement _ _ _ _ _

Feel the ebb and flow of energy as you breathe _ _ _ _ _

Each moment is different _ _ _ _ _

Each part of each second in time is different _ _ _ _ _

When your arm is finally on the floor_ _ _ _ _ rest and relax for a few minutes. *(Allow 2–3 minutes for this)*

Now bring your attention to your left arm _ _ _ _ _ and prepare to repeat the exercise _ _ _ _ _

Breathe in and lift to the vertical _ _ _ _ _ allowing about 2½ minutes, keep breathing gently and in your own time, but taking about 2½ minutes _ _ _ _ _

Breathe out and begin to *slowly* lower it _ _ _ _ _

Maintain your concentration on your left arm _ _ _ _ _

On your breathing _ _ _ _ _ at a steady rate _ _ _ _ _

To the energy being brought to your arm as you breathe in _ _ _ _ _

And the control as you lower it _ _ _ _ _

Breathing steadily all the time _ _ _ _ _

Bringing energy to the arm _ _ _ _ _

Don't speed up the movement as it becomes more difficult _ _ _ _ _

Keep concentrating on the moment _ _ _ _ _

Feel the air around it as you lower the arm _ _ _ _ _

Breathing gently and steadily _ _ _ _ _

If you find it uncomfortable _ _ _ _ _

Come back to your centre of stillness . . . . .

To your breathing _ _ _ _ _

Bringing energy to the arm _ _ _ _ _

Feel the floor seeming to move away from you slightly as you lower the arm _ _ _ _ _

Notice the difference in the sensations in the other parts of your body _ _ _ _ _

In the other arm _ _ _ _ _

Bring your attention back to your left arm, notice the ebb and flow of energy in the arm _ _ _ _ _

Each second is different _ _ _ _ _

Each moment is new and unique _ _ _ _ _

You will never feel exactly this moment again _ _ _ _ _

Breathing into the movement _ _ _ _ _

When your arm is finally on the floor, rest and relax your whole body _ _ _ _ _

Lie with both arms relaxed by your sides _ _ _ _ _

Breathing gently _ _ _ _ _

Feeling relaxed. *(Allow 2–3 minutes for this)*

Breathe in and raise both arms to the vertical . . . . .

And take them back to either side of your head or as far as you can . . . . .

Breathe out and lower them to your sides in one breath . . . . .

Rest . . . . .

This time breathe in . . . . .

Breathe out and raise your arms above your head . . . . .

Notice how unbalanced and strained the movement feels without the influx of air to sustain the energy . . . . .

Lower your arms to your sides . . . . .

Once again, to compare the movement . . . . .

Breathe in and lift the arms to either side of your head or as far as you can . . . . .

Breathe out and lower them . . . . .

This time breathe in, turn your hands palm upwards . . . . .

Lift the arms to the vertical with the palms turned upwards . . . . .

Breathe out and lower them down . . . . .

Notice how the movement feels to you . . . . .

Breathe in, and turn your hands plams down . . . . .

Lift the arms up to the vertical with the palms turned downwards
. . . . .

Compare this movement with the palm upward movement . . . . .

Notice what it does to *you* as an individual . . . . .

When the palms are turned upwards, the movement is open and supplicating. This is a universally understood gesture. When the palms are turned down, it is as though you are more oriented to the earth and the movement draws your hands regretfully away from it.

Lesson 14

Relaxation for insomnia

> Insomnia is not a disease or an attack by a virus. Sometimes insomnia may be symptomatic of disease but to the millions of otherwise healthy people who take sleeping tablets every night it is a functional disorder. If we cannot sleep it is because we have lost the art of sleeping. Drug-induced sleep is no cure for insomnia nor do the results have the same restorative effect as natural sleeping.
>
> Ursula Fleming, *The Desert and the Marketplace*

Editor's Introduction

This lesson can be taught in class or to individual patients who must remain in bed. Pillows may be used for the exercise as it creates a sense of comfort and realism in the class. Students can be assured that even though they may not fall asleep at first, practise will ensure success and that thinking about *not* sleeping will always make the situation worse.

The exercise for this lesson can be used following lessons 1 or 2 if the student has a long history of insomnia or is very stressed. Poor sleeping patterns are often the development of habits that prevent sleep. Anyone who cannot get to sleep or remain asleep should try to eliminate:
1.   Any form of mental stimulation before trying to go to sleep. This includes reading textbooks, reports or any other documents related to work, watching frightening or thought provoking television programmes, planning future activities – even holidays.
2.   Chemical stimulants including tea, coffee, cola, cigarettes and alcohol.
3.   Eating large or heavy meals ('night hunger' is a myth – your digestive system needs to rest).

Remember that it is the quality of sleep that is important, not so much the quantity. You can sleep for 9 hours tossing and turning and wake up feeling just as tired as when you went to bed, or you can sleep deeply and easily for 6 hours and feel fine.

Instructions for students

First of all, don't be afraid. Sleep will come if you let it. If you prefer, cover your eyes.

Relax your body as you have learned *(allow 2–3 minutes).*

Concentrate on breathing . . . . .

Raise your right forearm on to the elbow and let it fall . . . . .

Raise your left forearm on to the elbow and let it fall . . . . .

Raise your right knee and let it fall . . . . .

Raise your left knee and let it fall . . . . .

If your mind will not settle, try lying on the stick for a while. This helps to relax your body and bring your mind back into the present time without images, thoughts and expectations.

Breathe out deeply . . . . .

Feel your weight go down on to the floor . . . . .

Follow each breath deeper each time you breathe out . . . . .

Don't visualize . . . . .

Look into the darkness . . . . .

Let your head rest . . . . .

Relax your eyebrows and the muscles around your eyes . . . . .

Relax as though you can feel even your bones relaxing around your eyes . . . . .

Allow your eyes to soften . . . . .

Feel the difference as it happens . . . . .

Softening all around your eyes . . . . .

And in your eyes . . . . .

Feel the air entering as you breathe . . . . .

Follow the air as it enters your face . . . . .

Follow it as it comes into your head . . . . .

Let it go right into the farthest reaches of your head . . . . .

As if it is cleaning it . . . . .

Feel the back of your head on the pillow . . . . .

Feel the muscles in the back of your head and neck relaxing . . . . .

Follow your breathing into the muscles of your head . . . . .

Feel them softening . . . . . relaxing . . . . .

Come back to your breathing . . . . . feel how shallow it is . . . . . how relaxed it is . . . . .

Feel the ebb and flow of your breathing . . . . .

Extend your breathing into your arms and legs . . . . .

Lift your arms and let them fall . . . . .

Lift them with the swell of your breathing . . . . .

Notice, as you breathe in, your arm becomes lighter before you lift it . . . . .

Really feel that lightness as you breathe in . . . . .

Become enfolded by a feeling of lightness . . . . .

Feel the pull of gravity as you become lighter . . . . .

Feel the lightness pulling you away from the earth as you breathe in . . . . . letting you gently back down as you breathe out . . . . .

Feel as though you are landing on a large soft cushion . . . . .

Before you open your eyes, stretch, turn on to your side and sit up before standing up.

Teaching the Fleming Method to patients with specific needs and problems

by Carol Horrigan

Assessment of a patient or group participants

All patients will have had a medical, physiotherapy or nursing assessment carried out before beginning to learn to use the Fleming Method. In some departments and health authorities the teacher may also be required to obtain permission from the doctor in charge of the case – or, for the mentally frail patient, from a carer. This is vitally important for the patient's safety, and a sensible precaution for the teacher in view of the potential for litigation from any injuries which may be ascribed to the use of the Fleming Method. It is a wise precaution to also ask each group of students embarking on a training class if they have any congenital or acquired deformities which may preclude them from carrying out the exercises without adaptation, or any health problems which they may believe to be exacerbated by exercise or lying on the floor. Assure them that very few people cannot participate in some way, and that the lessons will be amended for their comfort and abilities.

Teaching children

When teaching children under sixteen years of age, obtain permission from a parent or carer and always have an adult family member present throughout the lesson.

Patients who cannot lie down flat on the floor

Most of the lessons begin with the person lying on the floor. This is the easiest position in which to gain maximum initial relaxation. If lying down on the floor is difficult or impossible however, do not force the patient to do so or let them think that they are not going to be able to use the technique as effectively as someone who can. Adapt their posture to a comfortable sitting or semi-recumbent position with all their limbs and head well supported, and they will be able to learn the method in their own way and at their own pace.

People with breathing difficulties

Diseases that affect normal respiratory function or requiring the use of tracheostomy may prevent the initiation of the technique lying down. For people experiencing these difficulties, an upright position will aid their remaining function and allow them to begin to use the technique. Impaired respiratory function could appear to be a major problem when learning the technique because observation of normal breathing patterns, and being able to use the breath as a controlling mechanism, are crucial for success.This does not preclude the use of the technique for such patients. Although they may take a little longer to feel confident, they will find they are able to gain control and alleviate the feeling of panic which often accompanies difficult or painful breathing. Patients with asthma should learn the technique when they are well so that they can apply it as soon as an attack starts and before it becomes a serious problem. The relaxation technique is *not* a cure for their disease process, but it can help overcome panic, and can help with control of both the frequency and severity of attacks.

> **NB: Always advise asthma patients that they must not discard their medication and should always carry their inhaler as usual. Only their doctor can advise them when to stop taking oral medication and inhalers which are prescribed for the prevention and control of attacks. They may find, however, that they need to use inhalers intended to be used during attacks less frequently.**

People with limb/joint pain or deformity

Amputees or those suffering with limb problems such as rheumatoid arthritis will also require an adapted technique. This will entail changing the scripts, paying particular attention to movements they may not be able to achieve. Patients may become embarrassed or physically distressed, and it is important that the therapist demonstrates an ability to create an individualized script related to each patient's needs when teaching a technique that could so profoundly change their outlook on symptom control. The patient with rheumatoid or other types of arthritis will need to move more frequently at first when learning the technique, because their joints can become stiff and 'locked' if they stay in one position for more than a few minutes. They may also have to use pillows or rolled, soft towels to support their joints during the sessions. Lying flat on the floor will almost certainly be an impossibility for many of them.

The technique can be adapted for patients who use a wheelchair. They may take a little longer to attain the feeling of relaxation, but the final outcome will be the same (see Case Histories).

People with learning difficulties

The scripts should be adapted by the teachers or nurses who are caring for the group or individual using appropriately adjusted language. The words and phrases of the original scripts can be changed to aid comprehension and, if necessary, shortened to fit the individual or group's attention span. If you do not have specialist training in this area and would like to use the method with someone who has learning difficulties, consult their relatives, usual teacher or therapist/nurse. They will be able to advise you on vocabulary, or idiosyncrasies of comprehension that they usually make allowances for. This will not only enable the patient to learn the method more effectively, but it will reduce the risks of embarrassing, frustrating and possibly overtiring someone already experiencing difficulties with learning new information or who is weakened by concurrent physical illness.

Surgical patients

Ursula Fleming's observations on teaching patients undergoing surgery

Ursula Fleming believed that, if at all possible, patients should learn the method before going to the operating theatre. She advocated a domiciliary visit at this time to teach the patient relaxation for pain control, and if the time scale allowed only one visit, a tape recording of the method could be left with the patient to practise further before admission to hospital. She felt this was better than attempting to teach the patient while nurses and doctors were trying to do their part before the operation and practising relaxation might be seen as an extraneous matter and disregarded by the patient and staff alike.

She preferred to visit the patient as soon as possible postoperatively, in the ward or intensive care unit. It was her observation that patients were, in most cases, unwilling to use a tape in the immediate postoperative period. She gave several reasons for this. A patient's locus of control is limited after surgery by discomfort such as pain, nausea or sleepiness. They expect and receive chemical pain and other symptom control provided by the medical and nursing staff, which is standard care and vital for recovery to proceed smoothly. Also patients find it hard to make decisions when they are still partially under the combined effects of anaesthetic and analgesic agents and manipulating a machine, however simple, can become just too taxing after surgery. She reported returning to patients who said the cassette recorder was malfunctioning only to find they simply hadn't re-wound the tape.

She found that some patients would listen to a tape before surgery but found this unnecessary postoperatively because the exercises were easy to learn and they could use them from memory. Patients in the recovery room often try to remove their oxygen masks, and headphones at this stage would be an added irritant. Therefore, for all these reasons, Ursula Fleming believed the use of tape recordings was best confined to the preoperative period.

By the time she saw them again on the ward postoperatively, patients' motivation to recover some of their locus of control was usually very high and they were able to concentrate more on the technique. Their level of anxiety would remain high for several days as they speculated about their future, their reactions, the possibility of pain, removal of sutures, and many other things. She felt that patients who did not admit to any anxiety were probably denying it for reasons of their own. As the therapist/teacher, she was interested in how they coped with this anxiety and whether, in the short time in which she saw them, she had been able to help stop the anxiety from exacerbating their pain.

Pain control

The following text is adapted from an article by Ursula Fleming published in the *Journal of Orthopaedic Medicine* (1988), No.1, 21–30.

The Fleming method of pain control is a psycho-physiological means of teaching patients to increase their level of pain tolerance.

The physiological effects aimed at are:

1. Release of habitual muscular tension.
2. Control of muscle spasm.
3. Increased mobility by coordinating movement with breathing.
4. Correcting faulty posture.

The psychological effects aimed at are:

1. Increasing the ability of the individual to focus their attention.
2. To control (not inhibit) emotion.

Prior to and following surgery may be an excruciatingly painful time. Remaining in a constant state of muscular tension in order to protect themselves from further pain can become so habitual that patients are frequently unaware of what it might feel like to be relaxed again. Learning to relax preoperatively by (if possible) lying flat on a hard surface increases awareness of tension. Without that awareness, it is impossible for patients to learn to 'relax themselves'. Lying in this position also helps to modify adopted postural defects, such as arching the spine away from back pain. The support offered by the floor also enables patients to relax completely and slow their rate of breathing.

Control of muscle spasm
When patients feel muscles beginning to tighten before they actually develop spasm they should:

1. Stop all movement.
2. Focus attention on the muscular tension and then let it go. This controls the tendency to panic.
3. Breathe *out* deeply.

Increasing mobility
In attempting to protect themselves from pain, patients often mobilize in strange, inefficient ways, for example, turning on to one side and pulling up with the arms, thereby increasing the strain on the back even when the need for such protection is no longer there.

Postoperative patients frequently attempt to get up from bed and reach the chair they want to sit in, holding their breath throughout the movement.

Staging movement
Getting out of bed can be divided into three stages:
1. Turning on to the side
   (a) Relax while lying flat and focus on calm breathing.
   (b) Breathe in deeply and simultaneously turn with the umbilicus forward. If possible, stretch up with the arm on to which the patient has rolled.
2. Sitting up
   (a) Relax in stillness and calm the breathing.
   (b) Breathe in deeply and, simultaneously push down with the uppermost arm to the sitting position. Ease the legs over the edge of the bed.
   (c) Rest and calm the breathing again.
3. From sitting to standing
   (a) Calm the breathing.
   (b) Breathe in and simultaneously transfer the weight to the feet and stand up.
   (c) Rest, relax again and calm the breathing.

Correcting faulty posture
Encourage patients not to sit with the spine curving backwards (see Figure 1, p. 65). If the head is thrust forward and the spine is curved, breathing is impaired by the compression of the abdominal organs upwards into the

thoracic cavity, and tensions in the muscle increase in proportion to their original pain (i.e. the amount of 'guarding' they are doing to prevent further pain), and how long they have been sitting in that position. Correcting posture can lead to an almost immediate diminution of the pain.

[Editor's note: Correct posture and therefore improved lung expansion reduces the risk of postoperative respiratory infection, improves oxygenation of tissues and potentially improves wound healing.]

Increased ability to focus attention
The patient should concentrate on immediate sensory input, allowing no speculation as to past or future connections. This is in a way learning to bypass the mechanical, discursive thinking which occupies so much of our mental energy and which can stimulate an emotional response relating not only to the immediate situation, based on past experience, but to all the future predictions of what that situation might lead to. In using the method this is firmly defined as 'fantasy' – a product of the imagination.

To focus the attention in this way lessens an emotional response to postoperative sensations which may be fuelled by fantasy.

The ability to control (not to inhibit) emotion
Conditioning In our society, relief from pain is seen as a right and a necessity. Pain is not evil; without it humans would not survive. People born congenitally insensitive to pain wreak the most horrific injuries on their own bodies without knowing it. The trouble with seeing pain as a malevolent attack from some external source is that frequently the resulting response to it is beyond the individual's locus of control and the patient fights rather than tolerates it and this engenders panic.

In this therapy, the patients are taught to recognize their instinctive recoil from pain (sometimes even before it happens or when it does, as at the dentist, when the known result will be curative), and to relax and accept it instead.

Emotional control Physical and physiological changes are often noted by the emotional changes that occur simultaneously. Conversely, emotional stress can cause physiological changes to take place. Melzack and Wall suggest that in pain 'messages from the spinal cord can be changed by messages coming down from the brain' and that 'these downward influences include the cognitive and other psychological factors such as anxiety and anticipation'.

The main factor to be avoided if acute pain is to be controlled is the onset of panic. Such control is not achieved by 'will-power' or by 'fighting', because these build tension, but by changing the physiological pattern which is either set up by or follows the onset of an emotion – by reacting not with tension but with relaxation.

1. Stop all movement.
2. Breathe *out* deeply.
3. Relax the areas where a sympathetic tension has built up, for example the teeth are clenched, the fists are tightened, or the eyes are hardened.
4. Focus on each sensory experience without letting the imagination change them into something other than what they really are.

[Editor's note: The greatest healer is relaxed sleep. Allowing and indeed encouraging patients to sleep naturally following anaesthesia is a gift to them. They may consider that they have to be alert, sitting up and entertaining their visitors a few hours following an operation, but their recovery will be consolidated and swifter if their bodies are allowed to follow their own inclination to recuperate from the onslaught of the chemical and physical interventions of surgery.]

If they are having difficulties in returning to a restful sleep, take them through the routine for insomnia described on pp. 94–6.

The person with chronic pain

All the basic principles of the Fleming Method apply to helping those who suffer chronic pain. Such people may not be patients in the sense that they are no longer in active orthodox therapy except for taking prescribed analgesics. They may live every day with pain as a constant and unwelcome companion and yet only call upon their doctor or community nurse if their symptoms change.

The Fleming Method can be used to train a person in pain to reverse their instinctive behaviour of tensing and to accept the pain, relaxing into it as a sensation. If they fight it, they will exacerbate the pain. When a person has been in pain for a considerable time, the problems become interpersonal as well as individual: their pain affects everyone who comes into contact with them. It must be a great temptation – and it may not be a conscious act – for the person in pain to use their suffering as a means of manipulating others. Equally, those others may suspect such manipulation, even when nothing of the sort was or is intended. Persistent pain has a depressing, defeating effect, and the patient may feel both resentful and guilty at the same time.

Here the therapist has to deal with both the physical and the underlying, sometimes unrecognized, emotional pain as well. Anything which motivates the person to take control lessens the sense of defeat. Therefore, alongside learning to use the Fleming Method, the student should be encouraged to use planning diaries, and to chart daily progress of achievements. All of these can help to control the tension, whether generated by depression or by an habitual reaction to the pain itself, which in turn exacerbates pain.

Measuring pain is always difficult; there is no objective means by which a patient can evaluate levels of pain. It may be that in measuring the effects of relaxation therapy it is not the pain itself that should be measured but the person's ability to tolerate it. Thus it is the person's *complaints* about the pain which should perhaps be noted, not the other factors that researchers commonly attempt to measure, such as duration, type, severity, onset and so on.

The objective of the therapy is, at all times, to accept rather than reject painful sensations. In labour, for example – described by Melzack as the worst pain – the intensity of the contractions, and therefore the pain, increases but the level of tolerance to the pain will be unchanged unless the patient relaxes and accepts it.

The care of mental health patients

> I am very grateful to the psychiatrists under whom I worked in my training and from whom I learned 'If you cannot do any good, make sure that you don't do any harm'.
>
> Ursula Fleming

Ursula Fleming spent several years working alongside the doctors, nurses and psychotherapists of the psychiatric unit at the Crichton Royal Hospital, Dumfries, Scotland. Here she observed orthodox methods of treating mental illness, and was able to work under medical supervision as a relaxation therapist. She displayed great insight into the patients' problems and empathy for them as individuals. The following section, adapted from her own writing, illustrates her philosophy in working with them using relaxation.

Teaching patients who are mentally ill

One of the values of this method of relaxation is that patients with mental health problems are able to use it to achieve greater perception about themselves and their condition. In conversations with patients who were diagnosed as having 'schizophrenia', some were beginning to be able to recognize the onset of an acute episode, and given appropriate help, they were able to avert the worst of the symptoms.

It is important that patients are not encouraged to fantasize even when they do not have mental illness. When they learn the Fleming Method, imagery is most definitely discouraged. It can be useful at times, but not for patients who are already experiencing auditory, olfactory or visual hallucinations. In our everyday living we often fantasize, but the main emphasis of this discipline is to train yourself to come to grips with reality. There can be great happiness and ineffable magic in reality itself, but fantasy is only a product of the mind and if the mind is in any way malfunctioning, fantasy can become a threatening and dangerous disturbance.

If patients say in the first lesson that they feel as though they are floating in space, always assure them that they are not. During all the lessons they are very securely grounded. If they doubt it, ask them to lie on a stick for a while to bring them back to reality. The discomfort of the stick, and the teacher's practical tone of voice, is sufficient to bring them back down to earth.

This is where, as a teacher, you have to be enormously honest. It is a temptation to encourage everyone to have a lovely time floating around in some imaginary limbo, but it will not help them. It is far more valuable to become immersed in the here and now, in this moment of time, and this dimension of space and no other.

Patients suffering from anxiety states are always over-tense and breathe inappropriately. Medication will always alleviate their symptoms and this is comforting to them, but it doesn't tackle the *cause* of the symptoms. Sometimes psychotherapy, talking out their problems, brings about an abreaction, some long-forgotten hurt is remembered, released or challenged and the patient is liberated.

Learning relaxation can help patients who are going through this process and experience. Any anxiety is manifest by tension in breathing; if patients learn to calm their breathing patterns then they will begin to gain confidence that their condition is not wholly beyond their control.

The despair and, for some, the feeling of humiliation, suffered when psychiatric help is needed to cope with life, cannot be imagined by anyone who has not personally experienced it. Anything which proves to them that they can have the power to control their own symptoms is immediately beneficial.

It is important to aim at small things first. After the first session there will always be questions. Patients must be assured that your voice has nothing to do with their ability to use the method, although they have responded to you and the words you used, it is *they* themselves who were able to relax. They just listened to instructions and followed them to the conclusion – a relaxed state. Be confident when you assure them that, indeed, they *will* be able to do it by themselves, even though some may rely on the teacher for a long time. It is essential that they practise on their own.

During the time that patients are learning to be independent with the method, they will reach a 'plateau of learning', where they seem to have reached a final level of relaxation beyond which they cannot go. The first sessions bring dramatic improvements, and then there may be a long pause where no improvement appears to be made, that is until there is another release which precipitates a great jump forward. With patients who are mentally ill (although it can happen to patients with physical illness), such a release can bring about an abreaction. They can become very upset, remembering something long-forgotten, but then the tension is eased and new depths of relaxation can be achieved. The teacher must be aware of this in group sessions, and observe every individual for the signs. Sometimes you may need to finish a session early and disband the group in order to give full attention to the one person who needs it. Timing is of the essence, and full professional support must be given to any patient who is obviously working through something which is difficult for them.

Sometimes a patient will want to be left alone in a state of tension even though it is painful. If it is giving them protection from the reality which is still too agonizing to face, only the patient can decide when the time is right to change. The teacher must tread very gently in situations like this, and make sure that the burden of truth is not too great to bear at that time.

Case Histories

Informal case notes

by Ursula Fleming

Editor's Introduction

Ursula Fleming recorded her observations and details of each training session directly into patients' case notes. All patients differ markedly in their reactions to training in the method and its effects. Occasionally their reactions were quite bizarre, demanding sensitive responses from the teacher. Some of Ursula's patients moved her so deeply that she also wrote about them in her day books. The entries were undated and she always used pseudonyms. Most of the patients described in the notes that follow were referred to her because orthodox prescriptions alone were unable to control their pain and abate their anxiety. In her writings Ursula laid bare the emotions that these patients engendered in her, how she planned further sessions and how she gauged her own successes and failures. In this she once again demonstrated how she was thirty years ahead of her time in working as a truly reflective practitioner. In the 1990s nurses have only just begun to use reflection seriously as part of their mandate.

Here are just some of her thoughts and hopes, her frustrations and her honesty, presented always with her patients' best interests at heart. Often she would maintain her visits after the patient had learned the method well. Sometimes, just as nurses become involved with a family, Ursula would too. Although she viewed the patient as the most important part of 'the team', she never forgot that illness affects all of those who are close to the patient and would often teach a partner to use relaxation as part of their own support mechanism. Even when her own health was failing, she continued to help others, strong in her belief that the empowerment of a person to control their own symptoms as much as possible was paramount to their quality of life.

Mr L...
Diagnosis: Large bowel partly obstructed by cancer

[Ursula did not indicate the number of days between visits]

Visit 1

This unfortunate man is very angry. The doctors have been honest with him about his diagnosis and the likely outcome. He is a comparatively young family man.

Visit 2
We have met on two occasions now and I have also left him some tapes. Today he complained of tension in the legs and feet and that the tapes were not long enough.

Visit 3
A long session today and for the first time he talked about himself. His doctor approved of this as he has been withdrawn. Seems he has always been so since he found that he had to work harder than anyone else to succeed at school.

Never had time to talk, or for hobbies, but grew to be successful as an adult. Enjoys talking about the economic situation. Without his job, he has nothing to occupy him and has become depressed. Talked about his children. He relaxed well – even his legs when he worked on them. Very twitchy but better eventually: said the pain never goes completely but it wasn't bad. Says he is 'scared witless' at the prospect of death and aware that he's missed a lot in his life because he concentrated on making his future secure. We talked about being absorbed in immediacy as the answer to fear of the future or regret for the past.

Visit 4
Readmitted with further acute obstruction but very happy – almost euphoric. His wife had brought him books and puzzles and these kept him occupied. Very kindly and helpful towards the deaf man in the next bed. Later he collapsed in great pain and had an emergency colostomy. I saw him the next day and he said, 'If ever I needed to relax it was then. And I could. I was able to reassure my wife that it would be alright. And it was. I don't really care if the colostomy is permanent or not.' No longer euphoric but his prognosis is very bad – only weeks not months to live according to his consultant. Very upset by the death of the patient in the next bed. Both he and his wife were united in this friendship and he also missed helping the old man.

Visit 5
Ten days after the colostomy he collapsed with a further obstruction. When I saw him he asked only to be 'put out' – 'I've had enough. I just want to go'. I stayed with him, working through the relaxation, getting him to trust in himself, making him let go of the tension. By the evening his recovery was dramatic and the colostomy was working. Both he and his wife ascribed this to the relaxation.

Visit 6
I haven't seen Mr L... for three days and he is visibly weaker with a poor colour. He asked me to work with him and he reacted very well. This was the best time of all, but I am worried that he is relying too much on me and not the technique. We talked about how he thought of the sensations in his body and he said 'in colour – when I relax I see deep purple and sometimes there are yellow edges like clouds. There are no colours when I am tense.'

Today after he relaxed I asked him how he felt. 'Peace. It's all peace. And there are banks and banks of flowers. I don't know where they come from.'

Visit 7
Mr L... and his wife resentful that I am going on holiday even though he is coping

well with the relaxation. I feel that the relationship is deteriorating but I think that this is a good thing. They had started calling me 'the angel of mercy' etc. which I find intensely embarrassing. Mr L... seems to be trying to make me feel guilty for not spending time with him, but I believe that beyond a certain stage emotional dependence on me cannot be helpful. Dying is a lonely business and that has to be faced. It is his family who need to share it with him. His wife asked me if she should bring their children to see their father for Christmas. We arranged that I would be with Mr L... to take him through the relaxation before they arrived. After his session he was very calm and the visit, the first from them since he had been admitted, went off very well. This made Mr L... very happy.

Visit 8
The ward Sister phoned a few days later to say that Mr L... had an embolus and was very scared. I stayed with him for two hours but there was only a slight improvement. 'It won't come,' he said, meaning the relaxation. I felt that he was blocking it somehow.

Visit 9
The next day he was asleep when I arrived but he had been practising on his own. I talked with his wife and she said that they both thought that I did him more good than all the medicines and treatments and asked me not to let up with him.

Visit 10
Today Mr L... told me that he had been very upset, thinking about why it should happen to him, and thinking about his family and being afraid. I told him about another patient who had 'died' during surgery and could remember being resuscitated. She was completely unafraid of dying afterwards. When we then went through the relaxation he was able to do it really well.

Visit 11
Mr L... had an unusual pain in a different area today and was maudlin and miserable, saying he knows that when he's down he upsets the nurses. Went back later and he had relaxed and was cheerful, reading the paper and even cracking jokes.

Visit 12
Today Mr L... told one of the nurses that I had 'lost' something, because although the relaxation still works, it gets harder to do. As I went into the ward he started a rigor. Relaxed him for a few minutes and he became warm again from being literally blue with cold. He said I had 'done the miracle again'.

Unfortunately, this was the most offputting thing he could say. I must sort out my attitude to this dependency.

From this point on Mr L... practised his relaxation every day and his wife and I were with him when he died. His leg had become very swollen and painful, he tried very hard with his relaxation until the last. The family invited me to the funeral. They gave me flowers and his brother thanked me for making his death easier.

Mrs A..., aged 45
Diagnosis: Breast cancer with metastases

[Visits to this patient were 2–3 days apart]

Visit 1
She is exceptionally tense. Her voice is appallingly flat and dead-sounding. Unable to remain still for more than one minute at the most. Clasping her hands and almost wringing them continually. Sitting and moving with her shoulders hunched, her whole body is set in a shell of protective tension. When she walks she takes tiny limping and shuffling steps across the floor; at rest she assumes an almost catatonic appearance.

Her body image is very bad, as if her body is an enemy to be hated and feared. She wears unattractive clothes in bright red and other clashing bright colours. Kubler-Ross considers the wearing of bright red signifies excessive pain and I think this is significant. This image only dates from her illness and enduring despair. Her house shows that by nature she is a craftswoman, very much engaged with balance of colour and shapes. A very 'visual' person. The clash in her clothing is like a scream for help – a signal to anyone who might listen, and very few do, that the pain of both body and mind are destroying her.

Her whole body coordination is poor, she takes no pleasure in it now. Preparing and eating food is totally dreary – deciding what to eat is a major problem and she feels guilty about this as it affects her family too.

She says that she feels 'safe' lying curled up in a fetal position on the sofa. She is bitter and resentful, feels that there is no one she can turn to for comfort and that she is sliding inevitably towards death. Separated from her husband, she worries constantly about her children and whether they will achieve the academic goals that she has set for them. Very fond of them but gains no comfort from them.

Mrs A... is completely lonely and withdrawn, so emotionally cold that it is almost frightening. Understandably, she is aggressive and suspicious because she felt no one believed her side of the separation story, that she was the innocent party. Rejects home visits from the nurse – 'she doesn't do anything'.

First relaxation session carried out on the sofa – could not lie on the floor. Gradually relaxed and lay comfortably. Fairly negative – 'Yes it feels better but you can't be here all the time and I won't be able to do it on my own.' I said 'Wait and see.'

Visit 2
Appears much better. This is very significant and optimistic as she has obviously been thinking about how she exacerbates her own pain and insomnia by remaining so tense. Lay quietly on the sofa without jumping up and really 'let go'. As she is so visual I talked to her about seeing and relaxing her eyes much earlier than I usually bring this up. She said that she was so tense that she only saw her fear, but when I talked to her about 'softening' her eyes she was able to do so and, as a consquence, her whole face and head became more peaceful. Got her to catch a ball. At first her coordination was so bad that she could not catch it. But by relaxing her hands and eyes she could. She realized the significance of this and how it showed that she could control her own tension.

Visit 3

The most significant thing is that her eyes have softened – not so brittle or negative. Said that she had tried the 'seeing' exercise on her own and that because it had worked, she had felt her depression had eased. She allowed that she felt better but could not stop worrying about her son not working hard enough for his 'A' levels. We discussed the ineffectiveness of nagging at teenage children and that it only made everyone feel guilty and unhappy. When I left she stood at the door until the car was out of sight and from then onwards she did this every time.

Visit 4

Mrs A... doing well; she has been out. We tried out the relaxing through breathing exercise and it worked. Talked of her pride in her eldest son at university, but how anxious she is about the youngest going abroad on a school trip. I talked about how the tension of her anxieties was adding to the problems that were already there.

Visit 5

Mrs A... had slept badly because of the discomfort but had relaxed and stayed contentedly in bed until she went back to sleep. A big improvement. I left her giving me a big smile.

Visit 6

Said she uses the breathing a lot now, especially to control her tensions when cooking, which she hates.

Visit 7

Anxious again today following a deep discussion with a relative about how much she had changed. We talked about how illness can affect self-confidence but that in time it can gradually be built up again. Finds it intolerable when she is alone in the house with only her fear for company. She now takes her dog out for walks around the village. She said that the relaxation almost always works and she is very pleased with her improvement.

Mrs B..., aged 63
Diagnosis: Advanced cancer

Visit 1

Mrs B... is a widowed, retired nursing sister. Her worst fear is of losing her independence. Complained of weakness and lethargy. Talked about the shock effect of being told a day after undergoing a cholecystectomy that she had irreversible cancer. Had kept it 'bottled up – it's my way'. She resents the loss of activity and thinks that it is permanent, which isn't necessarily so. Says that she has no quality of life – just sitting and watching television. Encouraged her to sit on an upright chair with padding for her back and she found it more comfortable. Did no relaxation – just talked. Heard of her skill at embroidery and she said that she felt brighter for my coming. Doctor says she is dying of despair.

I feel like David with Saul.

Visit 2 [Two weeks later]
Started relaxation. I bought a small piece of embroidery and asked for her help in doing it. She became irritated by my ignorance – a good sign. Got up and went to communion. Talked about her grief for her husband; said she only felt half alive since he died twelve years ago. Says she would like to 'turn over and die'. Talked some more, and she has remembered all that we did in the first session. Maybe she will climb on my back till her own vitality returns.

Visit 3 [Next day]
Said she would surprise us by her improvement when I return in three days time. More positive. Ward Sister reported her improvement to the doctor.

Visit 4 [Next day]
Asleep – apparently.

Visit 5 [Three days later]
Doctor thinks that her improvement is not significant as she still needs help to get up etc. She requested physiotherapy to help her with her walking. Did relaxation but became irritable when we got to the breathing exercise. I think that the weekend break was too long; she still needs the support.

Visit 6 [Next day]
Complained of shortness of breath when doing physio. Walking better. Said that she wasn't trying hard enough, but didn't believe that she was being hysterical. Asked to see her doctor – if he gives her a date of discharge she feels that she would be able to make more effort.

Visit 7 (Two days later]
'I'll surprise you all one day' ... and yes she is better.

Visit 8 [Five days later]
A bad day. Pretended to be asleep when I arrived. No improvement. Very confused. I helped her to dress and go to the loo. Fell backwards and called for my help. There is something wrong with her speech – is this due to a change in her medication?

Visit 9 [Next day]
Very different. Bright. Looking forward to seeing me. Asked for my help in walking. Said that she must now make an effort or she could just 'wander off'. Very relieved mentally from the anxiety that the pain was from secondaries after the Consultant reassured her.
   Thanked me for helping her through such a difficult time.

Visit 10 [Next day]
Anxious when starting to walk. Very tense and shaking. Leaning forward and shuffling to begin and then able to hold her head up and look forward. Very cooperative and her walking improved during the visit. I left her sitting in a chair, said she would go back to bed for a sleep later.

Visit 11 [Two days later]
Great improvement.

Visit 12 [Twelve days later]
Despair. None of her relatives will let her stay with them to convalesce. They don't want the responsibility. Walking worse than ever. Talked for a while, then relaxed her and then walked with her again: '... head up ... breathe ... put your weight solidly on each foot ... don't shuffle ...'. Walked fine because she was relaxed.
    Gave her a tape to help her to sleep.

Visit 13 [Next day]
Verdict on the tape: 'Excellent!' Walking better. Very sunny so we went outside – the first time she had been out for eleven weeks. Talked about the possibility of living in a flat with a warden. Asked me to buy an audiotape as she had enjoyed listening to the one that I had lent her. I must watch out for overdependency.

Visit 14 [Next day]
Used the breathing exercise to help her get up. Walked much better today, out in the sun again. Talked about the ideal of having a loving husband to care for her or a sister, but her sisters were no longer alive either.

Visit 15 [Twelve days later]
In tears after seeing a doctor who told her that there was nothing else to be done. Another doctor told her that it wasn't so that 'everything had been tried', yet another congratulated her on her walking and wasn't in the least discouraging. That night she slept for twelve hours – feeling very depressed.

Visit 16 [Eight days later]
It has been arranged that Mrs B... be transferred to a hospital nearer to her relatives and where they can provide more physiotherapy. Apprehensive but also excited. Said she knows that she can do more.
    Left complaining slightly about the staff. To ease the parting from them?

Mr A..., aged 30
Diagnosis: Terminal cancer

Visit 1
Mr A... is married and the couple have two children. He looks very young. Quiet and polite – too polite. Very cooperative but left me feeling uneasy. Apparently he had been very disturbed by his prognosis before this admission. Sees the value of relaxing. Did it – apparently very well.

Visit 2 [One month later]
Very good relaxation – said he felt 'at peace'.
    But too quiet.

Visit 3 [Next day]
Said he'd had a good night. Left him with the tape recording of today's session.

Visit 4 [Next day]
Hadn't liked listening to the tape − had a bad night. Sat in a wheelchair for the first time in three weeks. Tired afterwards and relaxed very well. Said his pain had gone and he slept for an hour. Claims that if he wakes in the night he can relax the pain away without calling for analgesics.

Visit 5 [Four days later]
Depressed, and said his main trouble was his mental state. Talked to him and made him breathe in. As with many depressed people, he was breathing out too heavily. Said it helped.

Visit 6 [Six days later]
Said he needed to structure his day − that it frightened him to have no timetable. So we made a timetable which he then kept to as rigidly as possible. Doing well and has many people helping him. Decided to fade out.

Visit 7 [Twenty-five days later]
Mr A... had asked to see me. He had been at home but on the first day had begun to panic and had returned to the hospital. He said he had tachycardia and was dying of fright. When I arrived he was asking the staff to kill him. Hitting his arms against the bed and shouting that he wanted 'to die now, NOW!'. It seemed to me that he was acting like a petulant child, but he relaxed well. I went home but when I got there I started thinking about his mother. I had met her on my way out, and I began to think about how I would feel if it were my son. So I went back.

As I arrived he had begun the shouting again. A hastily convened and necessarily brief case conference with the nurses and the doctor brought the decision to keep him awake but relaxed for fixed intervals (with me) during the day, and the nurses would then use medication to sedate him at night so that everyone could get some sleep.

Visit 8 [Next day]
I was there when Mr A... woke and he had reverted to his petulant childishness. Relaxed him and stayed with him while he listened to some music. He kept looking up to see if I was still there. He talked about his faith and then went back to doing the breathing exercises. The Consultant came to see him, waiting until the tape ended – admirable timing − and then talking calmly to Mr A... about his thoughts on suicide.

Visit 9 [Seven days later]
Same as before − but more difficult.

Visit 10 [Next day]
Bad again. Says he is 'a living vegetable'. We talked about his value in being who he is rather than what he could do. He didn't believe me when I told him that he could get up any time he wished. The doctor reassured him and he agreed to get up and go out in a wheelchair with his wife. Very tired and 'droopy' when he returned. Told the doctor that the side of his head was painful and his sedation was increased.

Seven days later Mr A... died in the afternoon.

I don't feel happy about this case. I feel that maybe I should have been more assertive with him from the beginning. He was very close to his mother; maybe he needed more firm support.

Miss A...
Diagnosis: Early breast cancer

Very enthusiastic to try relaxation. She had been to see faith healers and other therapists. First showed her how changing her posture could ease the pain in her neck. Continued with the neck movements. Continued relaxation on the couch and at first her eyelids were moving like castanets! After a while her eyes stilled and her breathing became more relaxed and deep. Asked her to breathe down into her abdomen and to feel the movement against my hand. I don't usually do this but it is obviously effective.

The room and the chairs in it are unsuitable. Ideally I would have liked to see her move. She is eminently suited to relaxation therapy, but there is nowhere to see her. I could have used the video camera to show her the posture problem, and used a stick to help her to cope with any pain she might have in the future.

Miss B...
Diagnosis: Advanced breast cancer
[Home visit referred from outpatient's clinic]

Visit 1
Very large, warm and enthusiastic lady. Difficult to stop her talking – says she is over-talkative when she is nervous. Eyelids flickering a lot but her body seemed reasonably relaxed. Said she realized that her damaged right side was tense. Couldn't relax that arm until I showed her how to. Left leg more tense than the right as it has arthritis. Did a drawing of how she sees her breathing. Next time we will try using the stick and some humming.

Visit 2 [Next day]
Has been practising but not getting very far. The arm movements are bad but improved with help. Relaxed but I don't think that she really understands what we are trying to achieve.

Visit 3 [Three weeks later]
This lady has learned all that she can about relaxation. She will not increase her understanding any further because she cannot stop chattering – very difficult for me.

Miss D...
Diagnosis: Advanced breast cancer, paraplegic

Visit 1
Very afraid. Waiting for bone scan results. The spasms in her legs are sometimes violent. Reassured when the result of the bone scan came and it was good. Then

relaxed very well, legs and hands stopped shaking. Helped her to sit more straight in the wheelchair and found it less painful.

Visits 2–6 [Three to five days apart]
Relaxation quite good, becoming evangelistic about relaxation. Feet now warm, euphoric about this!

Visit 7 [Next day]
Relaxation and 'seeing'. Fell asleep.

Visit 8 [Six days later]
Physio is improving her movement and she is including the breathing exercises to help her. As soon as she can get from bed to chair she can go home.

Visit 9 [Eight days later]
Felt bad as a result of the chemotherapy. Relaxed and her colour returned. She could feel tingling in her legs.
   Said, 'You know no one can take this (the ability to relax) away from me, but when I talk about it they all laugh at me.' She is obviously happier and using relaxation to help her sleep.

Visit 10 [Two days later]
Day of discharge. She can relax so that she doesn't feel the pain of her injections.

Visit 11 [Five days later – at home]
Very distressed, hot and sweating. 'I've lost it – I can't do it any more!' Has had a tough time adjusting to her paraplegia at home and is bad tempered with her family. Relaxed well and seemed very happy as a result.

Visit 12 [One month later – readmitted with fracture]
Bright but aggressive about her bedsores and to her family. Thinks the nurses are fed up with her. Good relaxation session, can feel tingling and warmth in her legs.

[Editor's note: Ursula made a further sixteen visits to Miss B... during the next three and a half months. In that time they used relaxation to help her with having blood taken, receiving a blood transfusion, pain in her mastectomy area, suture removal (instead of diazepam), during X-rays, and periods of sadness and depression.]

Mrs C...
Diagnosis: Carcinomatosis
[Referred by her doctor]

Visit 1
Mrs C... is very pale, listless and she needs to learn relaxation to help her control vomiting. Relaxed well.

Visit 2 [Next day]
No vomiting for twenty-four hours. No more anti-emetics. Very good at relaxation; has practised on her own.

[Editor's note: Ursula made six more visits to Mrs C... in the next three weeks and recorded she was always very good at relaxing, even when death was approaching.]

Mrs D...
Diagnosis: Cancer

I have made several attempts with this lady but I cannot seem to get her to understand the concept of self-help. She cannot seem to concentrate or stop talking about other things.

Mrs E...
Diagnosis: Breast cancer with possible bone and liver involvement

Visit 1
First visited Mrs E... at her home. Devoted husband. In the beginning she found relaxing strange. Said that she felt self-conscious and was despondent about it.

Visit 2 [Seven days later]
Breast lump less angry. Relaxed well and we were both more positive.

[Editor's note: Ursula visited Mrs E... seven times, both in hospital and at home, in the following three and a half months, during which time Mrs E... used relaxation successfully on each occasion and when she was alone. Six weeks before Mrs E... died, Ursula recorded the following comments.]

Visit 10
Home visit. Less anxious to relax, wanted more to talk. I let this develop, and I think retrospectively it was a mistake.

Visit 11
From here on until her death, I saw her each day that I was on the ward. I was there to relieve her husband and to hold her before she died. I didn't relax her then because I felt that she didn't want it. Now I think that I was mistaken.

Mrs F...
Diagnosis: Cancer

Visit 1 [Home visit]
Very nervous woman. Anxious to see me and to fit in with my timing. Feels guilty that she hasn't been able to control her illness. Has been using the Simonton method. 'If it's wolves it's good because they get all the bad cells, they are more thorough, but if it's sharks it isn't so good – they might miss some.' [See Editor's notes on the Simonton method of visualization at the end of this case history.]

I taught her to relax without visualizing and she was very good. Mrs F... walks and sits with discomfort. She learned how to sit with her weight away from the coccyx, and to walk without putting her weight on her heels. The pain became easier and her movements much less stiff. Seemed very happy.

After only two more sessions, each seven days apart, Mrs F... reported that she could now walk, sit and lie down without any pain and that she felt much more positive.

[Editor's note: The Simonton technique uses visualization to maintain a positive attitude towards the body's own defence systems and towards medication, such as chemotherapy, and their respective abilities to destroy cancer cells. If the patient's health deteriorates, either because the tumour is very aggressive or chemotherapy was started when it was at an advanced stage, the patient may self-blame for their visualization abilities not being effective. They may believe (erroneously), that they have carried it out incorrectly or too infrequently. I have used the technique with patients and they have found it useful, but patients undertaking the technique should be counselled before they begin to use the method. Ideally, the patient, their relatives and the therapist should all have an honest opinion from the doctor regarding the status of the tumour. Although, at the present time, doctors will not be able to make an absolute statement as to the likelihood of any patient's survival, they can prevent much despair from a patient attempting such therapy when the indications are that it would be futile, and serve only to make the patient and everyone else involved feel guilty.]

Mrs G...
Diagnosis: Diabetes, breast cancer
[Referred from ward round]

Visit 1
Mrs G... is seriously overweight and her diabetes is not controlled. She has been warned by the medical staff about the effects of over-eating.

We talked about using simple will-power to stop the immediate need to eat and then to concentrate on the painful sensations of hunger and to breathe through them. Once she had gained control then she would divert her attention by doing a puzzle or something else with her hands. Relaxed well.

Visit 2 [Six days later]
Has been practising on her own, with success.

Visits 3–7 [Over nine days]
Doing well.

Visit 10 [Five days later]
Mrs G...'s arm is painful. Talked about accepting pain rather than rejecting it, and breathing through it etc. Very good at doing this.

Visit 11 and 12 [Two and four days later]
Coping well, very good at all the techniques she has learned. Says that they have helped more than anything in the past twelve years.

Mrs J...
Diagnosis: Advanced breast cancer

Visit 1
Immediately understood the method. Relaxed very well and wanted to know all about the practical applications of the method. Left her a tape.

Visit 2 [Six days later]
Had used the tape twice and each time had fallen asleep. As insomnia is one of her problems because of the persistent itching of her skin, this was a good start. She was itching at the moment and so we tested the effectiveness of the relaxation. After ten minutes the itch was gone and she was comfortable. She found this difficult to credit but could not deny it.

Visit 3 [Four weeks later]
Mrs J... is very ill today but enthusiastic about relaxation. Asked me if she should continue to fight her illness and I said, 'Yes'. Relaxed her before she went to sleep for the night.

Visit 4 [Next day]
Had slept well and was bright and cheerful. Walked about the ward. Legs less swollen.

Visit 5 [Next day]
Relaxed well, said, 'I can do the breathing control really well now.' Has breathing difficulties mostly after her radiotherapy and after eating.

Visit 6 [Next day]
Both Mrs J... and I were encouraged by the Consultant during his round. Worried about her husband. Relaxed well, breathing much better. Went to sleep.

Visit 7 [Five days later]
Pneumonia, but breathing is good and she is content. Another patient is screaming all the time. I couldn't stand it if I were in Mrs J...'s position, yet she is remarkably tolerant about it.

Visit 8 [Two days later]
The other patient is still screeching, but Mrs J... is relaxed even though her breathing is now restricted. She said that she didn't mind dying, she was only concerned for her husband.

Two days later Mrs J... died peacefully.

Mrs K...
Diagnosis: Advanced cancer, difficulties with walking

Visit 1
A talkative woman who gave me a detailed history of her illnesses. Relaxed well, and started using breathing exercise to help her stand, balanced in a frame.

Visit 2 [Seven days later]
Walked without the frame, got her to hold her head up as she walked. Very cheerful and optimistic. Talked about returning to work.

Visit 3 [Seven days later]
Walking well, less stooped. Feels that she doesn't need the relaxation sessions any more.

Mrs K... was always complaining about 'the system' and how badly she had been treated throughout her illness. I feel that maybe I should collaborate with the cancer nurses who visit, and talk about the levels of sympathy that I offer.

Mrs H...
Diagnosis: Advanced breast cancer

Visit 1
Mrs H... has at last agreed to see me after several months of persuasion by the staff. Very difficult first session as the ward was unusually noisy.

Visit 2 [Two days later]
Feels unwell today, left her to rest.

Visit 3 [Eight days later]
Unable to let her arm fall – 'I can't do this, I've been holding myself and the family together for so long, I can't "let go"'. She became distressed so we finished the session.

I visited Mrs H... on and off for the next eight months while she gradually learned and used the method to help her through her anger and pain, sleeping difficulties and finally a pulmonary embolus. Even in her final week she improved her ability to use the method, but an unexpected cardiac arrest ended her life.

Mrs I...
Diagnosis: Post mastectomy

A married woman whose children all lived some distance away. Said she was anxious and tense because her husband did not have any feelings or understanding about her illness and she felt alone with it. Her husband was worried more about how he would cope after her death than how he would care for her on her return home.

I saw her every day and we talked about her going home and about joining a new club. Used relaxation well to control her pain, although it was getting worse. The nurses reported that she was able to talk to them more easily following my visits.

Slowly her strength diminished until her final day. When I called to see her she held my hand, looked up and said, 'Eeh, love'. She died at four in the afternoon.

Mrs Z...
Diagnosis: Advanced breast cancer

Visit 1
First visit was on the ward. Mrs Z... is only twenty-eight and very afraid. Had to be lifted into a sitting position by two nurses. Rigid and sweating profusely. Relaxed her using the usual procedure with movement of the arms but not the legs. Appears to be quite good but difficult to assess because she is so polite.

Visit 2 [Next day, at home]
I suggested that muscular wasting was contributing to her weakness. She said that she could not tell the difference between the cancer pain and muscular pain. We went through the neck exercises but I advised caution in practising them. Left her a tape to practise with.

Visit 3 [Next day]
Very frightened to move, shoulders hunched with tension. Talked about the tilt of the sacrum and did the sitting exercises with breathing. When she was lying down I showed her the long arm movement which relaxed her shoulders and neck. A good session, said she found it helpful. Her approach to me is bland but I feel an underlying tension, almost aggression.

Visit 4 [Two days later]
Showed me, with great excitement, how she can now sit up by herself. She had done this for the first time the previous night. Very happy and grateful. We talked about the anxiety caused by looking too far ahead and how to control it by taking each day at a time, even though it was tempting to plan holidays etc.

Visit 5 [Two days later]
Anxious to sit up unsupported but her neck was hurting. I promised to talk to the Consultant and that, in the meantime, she should take things slowly.

Visit 6 [Next day]
The Consultant said that she could exercise till it hurts! She thought that she had already done too much. Very good at the arm movements, but not the legs. Can still feel a knot of tension in her neck which she cannot relax.

Visits 7–11 [Over the next fifteen days]
During this time Mrs Z... had begun to use relaxation regularly each day. She misses it when her children are at home at weekends and she cannot find time. Found that she could use relaxation to stop her 'feeling sorry for herself', and it gave her a feeling of independence. Is now aware of areas of tension when she goes out for a walk and can control them.

Visit 12 [Next day]
Today I was tired. We talked about pain, did the breathing and aligned it to body movements. Not bad, but my fault that it wasn't better.

Visit 13 [Four days later]
Walked well with a frame.

Visit 14 [Next day]
Mrs Z... feeling very ill today with aches and pains. She is working hard at relaxation. Taught her the 'seeing' exercise.

Visits 15–18 [Over the next 10 days]
A difficult session as the youngest child is also ill. Felt that she had lost all the improvement of the last few weeks. This is because she is so distracted by her sick child, she cannot cope with both. Her husband is also fraught. Nevertheless sessions good and she relaxed well. Feels that she still has blocks of tension in her hips.

Visit 19 [Next day]
Her husband and child now better and she is able to concentrate on her relaxation. Very good and productive session, able to relax her neck well now.

Visit 20 [Next day]
A good session again, but hard work. Her Consultant says her latest test results are not good and her prognosis is now poor. She still cannot fully relax. Is this the result of the cancer itself? She feels that she still cannot get her hips to relax.

I have rarely got past her bland exterior except for one occasion when she exclaimed how she felt about her prognosis and used some, only slightly, stronger language than normal. I would like to see her emote more freely. One of her nurses said that she has had periods of crying and screaming but it didn't seem to help. I feel that she has built up a defensive shell to protect her from everyone who is treating her. Is she emotionally imprisoned from a long way back?

Visits 21–24 [Four days apart]
Returned to the ward for chemotherapy. Had a tough time. Uncomfortable, sweating and finally pain in her hips. Relaxed well with me and with a tape. Still needs a lot of reassurance. Has lost confidence in her ability to fight; we talked at length about her fear of death and pain. I did some exercises with her, pressing hard into her hand so that she relaxed against the pain but could still feel safe. On one occasion she became hysterical whilst a doctor attempted to take blood. Used the method with me and calmed down for him to take it.

Visits 25–33 [Every day]
On the ward round [Visit 25], Mrs Z... suddenly said that the relaxation didn't work! Her Consultant asked me to keep going anyway. Then she told me that she could feel the breath in her legs for the first time – is she saying this just to please me? She had a long talk to the House Officer about her death and she was quite relaxed afterwards.

Visits 34–36 [Every day]
Encouraged by the Consultant to use relaxation, but I also assured her that he would not let her die in pain as she had feared. She is going to make her will and

write goodbye letters to her husband and children. I agreed that the greatest gift she could give them would be to be unafraid of death. They would then live their own lives unafraid. She said that the relaxation helped enormously to help her to remain calm.

Visits 37–55 [Every day]
During this time Mrs Z... used relaxation to help her cope with an operation under local anaesthetic, more chemotherapy, a persistent, dry cough which kept her awake, more radiotherapy, breathing difficulties and panic attacks. At times she was ecstatic with her own skill in using the method.

The day before she died the Consultant called to request that I visit because Mrs Z... would not have morphine. Unfortunately, I was too late for that final visit. In the night Mrs Z... had died following a cardiac arrest.

Mrs J...
Diagnosis: Advanced breast cancer

Time between visits varied between one and seventeen days and on one occasion, when Mrs J... returned home, for twenty-three days.

Visit 1
Talked for quite a while before trying the method. She was anxious to begin because she had been using relaxation tapes and found that she could not become relaxed by using them. Very good session, was able to relax well.

Visits 2–6 [Two to fourteen days apart]
Very good, using a stick to experience pain and is already doing sitting and seeing with great success. Can now control her breathing and speed of talking by doing so. Wants to try to stop blushing by trying the method.

Visits 7–15 [Six to twenty-three days apart]
Finds relaxing in bed easier than on the floor. Uses it regularly. Talks to me about her problems, especially about arranging her own funeral, as she feels that her husband will not cope. Has told other patients to see me. Went with her to the funeral of Mrs Z...

Visit 16 [Four days later]
Had been distressed by Mrs Z...'s funeral. Made her aware of the imminence of her own death, but was trying not to think about it.

Visits 17–25 [Four to thirteen days apart]
Very good sessions, feeling better. Sad, but resigned. Used relaxation to have cystoscopy without anaesthetic and coped very well.

Visit 26 [Thirteen days later]
Is going on holiday. Says that she can only contemplate leaving the 'safety' of the hospital now that she can use relaxation to help her through her pain. She can cope without analgesics and is determined that her family are going to enjoy the

holiday. She looks beautiful. Serene. She has accepted the things that she cannot change and knows that she is going to die soon.

Visit 27 [Twelve days later]
Had a marvellous holiday. Very brown, and looks more beautiful than before, and her friends and family are all commenting upon this. Very serene, no pain until she returned. Once again commented that she only dared to go away because she had the relaxation technique to rely on.

Visit 28 [Next day]
Selective hepatic embolization under local anaesthetic. Used relaxation for the procedure and made a good recovery.

Visit 29 [Next day]
Good recovery maintained.

Visit 30 [Next day]
Has renal failure. Gravely ill.

Visit 31 [Next day]
When I arrived the nurses told me that Mrs J... died from renal failure early this morning.

Mrs K...
Diagnosis: Breast disease, claustrophobia and other phobias

Visit 1
She is agitated and has many social problems. Her symptoms are overt and I believe may be exaggerated. Tried relaxation and it worked well.

Visit 2 [Five days later in outpatients department]
Has not practised or tried any of my suggestions, although she professes that she is 'desperate for help'.

Visit 3 [Six days later]
Mrs K...'s general practitioner has given her tranquillizers; she needs to adjust the dose as she keeps falling asleep. Unwilling to make the journey to outpatients again. I believe that her symptoms are serving a purpose and that she still needs them.

Miss E...
Diagnosis: Breast cancer with metasteases
[Weekly visits]

Visit 1 [In outpatients department]
A young woman of only 35 who at first refused the doctors' offer to see me. Has been receiving psychoanalysis for ten years. Suspicious, aggressive and yet worried about her condition. Competition daunts her and she becomes frustrated and angry.

Posture very poor, long sagging spine and her head drooping like a tulip. Relaxed very well. Showed her how to cope with pain. Was able to balance a stick upright on her hand – concentration very good and stopped her interminable self-analysis.

Visit 2
Pain in her back relieved by relaxation – good session.

Visit 3
Maintaining improvement.

Visit 4
Much less aggressive. Good relaxation.

Visit 5
Talked about making a concentrated effort to reverse the negative attitude that had forever plagued her. She can either succumb to it or do something about it.

Visit 6
Punctual for the first time. Relaxed very well. Revealed factors about her past that she had begun to face with her analyst. They included her reasons for blocking out her emotions.

Visit 7
Punctual again. Getting more positive. For the first time she did not mention cancer or pain. Relaxed well. Says it is emotionally painful, like analysis was at the beginning. Unfortunately her relationship with her analyst is now very dependent and not exciting.

Visit 8
Can reduce her anxiety by relaxing. Feeling much better and relieved.

Visit 9
Distressed to find that as relaxation begins to work it makes her feel vulnerable. Also her relationship with her analyst must change.

Visit 10
Always punctual nowadays with no missed appointments. Talked about spontaneous regression of cancer. Believes that she decided when she was a teenager that she would die from cancer when she was older. (If that was so, and she could induce the illness, then is she able to reverse the process?) We talked about the positive things in her life. She is going on holiday tomorrow.

I have seen her weekly since her holiday and she remains stable and relaxed.

Mrs L...
Diagnosis: Breast cancer

Visit 1
Very defensive and 'bristly'. Has done some singing training and so she can

control her breathing well. Many regrets in her life. At first did not show much interest in learning the technique, but relaxed surprisingly well.

Visit 2 [Eight days later]
Surprised at the additional breathing control the technique gives her. Concentrated on doing it seated. Shoulders very tense and head posture is weak. Good relaxation.

Visit 3 [Eight days later]
Found another lump today. Talked about things that made her feel guilty. Unafraid of death as long as she was prepared and it wasn't painful. Often falls asleep during a session and anxiety high over potential return to work. In case she falls asleep there. She cannot afford to lose her job. Accepts that her anxiety and depression may be exacerbating her symptoms. I suggested that she practised relaxation at lunchtime to offset 'tiredness'.

Visit 4 [Five days later]
Good session. No red flush when she saw the Consultant. Reassured about the new lump. (Mrs L... is the third woman patient I have treated who has been able to control her red flushes by regular use of the technique and the Consultant now often asks specifically for them to be taught it for this reason.)

Visit 5 [Next day]
Feeling 'unutterably tired'.

Visit 6 [Ten days later]
Pleased to be home when I visited her there.

Visit 7 [Two days later]
Long session. Phantom sensations in mastectomy site, and her voice is permanently damaged by radiotherapy. Feels that she has nothing to live for as her body image is ruined. Her main hobby now is listening to music, as she has abandoned all her friends, but relaxation is successful.

Visit 8 [Three months later – re-admitted for more chemotherapy]
Still able to relax well although her deteriorating condition is apparent. Talked about being afraid of chemotherapy and its after-effects.

Visit 9 [Next day]
Had used relaxation before chemotherapy and had not had any sickness. Very pleased.

Visit 10 [Five days later at home]
Arm very swollen and she is constipated. Depressed by how ill she feels. Nurse advised a laxative cocktail that was effective.

Visit 11 [Thirteen days later – re-admitted]
Responded well to relaxation.

Visits 12–16 [Daily]
Using technique well. Relaxed before having a Hickman line inserted, but is worried that she might not be able to manage it with her swollen hand.

Visit 17 [Two months later]
Coping with Hickman line.

Visit 18 [Next day]
Is seeing a hypnotist who is returning next week. I will hold my sessions so that she is not confused.

Visit 19 [Seven days later]
In pain and very distressed. Relaxed for forty-five minutes. Feeling very much better.

Visit 20
Asks to see me but when I arrive always has a reason for saying that she now doesn't have the time.

Visit 21 [Ten days later]
Asked if she could see me more often.

Visit 22 [Next day]
Couldn't see me for a variety of reasons.

Visit 23 [Next day]
Very aggressive and accusatory to a doctor who was having difficulty taking blood from her tense arm. I relaxed her and it then took him about two minutes.

Visits 24–26 [Fourteen days later]
She continued to use the technique during my absence of two weeks. When I returned her deterioration was marked. She did not wish to be disturbed in any way and lay quietly until her peaceful death.

Mrs M...
Diagnosis: Back pain

Sharp pain exacerbated by any stressful intrusion, for example the noise from the ward vacuum cleaner. Understands the relationship between the pain and her tensions. Difficulty walking because of the pain. Taught her to breathe into the pain to relieve it.

Mrs N...
Diagnosis: Dyspnoea
[Four visits over twelve days]

Mrs N... was red in the face from anger about her disease and the exertion of breathing. Relaxed well and her colour improved considerably. Very apprehensive about forthcoming chemotherapy. Did not require oxygen if she used the technique to calm herself.

Mrs O...
Diagnosis: Nausea/ 'nerves'
[Four visits over six weeks]

Has been using meditation. Consultant suggested that she see me. Relaxed very well and controlled the nausea. Also used the method for relaxed walking and seeing.

Mr C...
Diagnosis: Tension
[Six visits over five weeks]

Referred by his Consultant. Very tense man who is a 'manager' at work. Extremely agitated on the first visit, could hardly lie down, with twitching and jerking of his body. Relaxed well and practised by himself to become very good at relaxing himself and controlling his tension.

Mrs P...
Diagnosis: New admission for mastectomy
[Five vists over twelve days]

Relaxed very well before surgery and was determined that 'this will see me through'. She made a dramatic recovery from her operation, cheerful and sitting up receiving visitors that same afternoon. Almost pain-free. Very grateful for being able to learn the method. Always relaxed and uses it at any appropriate moment. Twelve days after her surgery she was able to return home and attended for chemotherapy at a later date. I did not see her after her discharge but I hear that she is now back in full-time work.

Miss X...
Diagnosis: Breast cancer, manic depressive – treated by Librium
[Six visits over fourteen weeks]

Referred by ward Sister. Has recurrent nightmares. Relaxed well and said 'I feel marvellous' afterwards. Verbose and very enthusiastic – 'It's worth losing a breast just to find this!' Saw her each time in out-patients clinic and she continues to do well.

Mr D...
Diagnosis: Carcinoma of the bronchus

A retired, married man in his sixties, he had pain in his back and his chest and difficulties with his breathing. Responded immediately to the practice of relaxation. Learned to deepen breathing and to calm himself by doing so. Immediately felt the benefit to his breathing and the pain eased also. After his discharge I visited him each week at home. He progressed a lot with his relaxation and was able to do it well without me or a tape. Developed a chest infection over Christmas and did not recover.

Mrs Q...
Diagnosis: Paraplegic with advanced breast cancer

Visit 1
Nurses reported that this patient was 'very aggressive', but I believed that I could help. She has been working with a 'Simonton expert' [see p.120] and says she does not require any further help.

Visit 2 [Two months later]
Again requested by nurses to see this patient who was reported to be in great pain. She still says that she puts all her faith in her psychotherapist, although he has now given up using the Simonton technique.

Visit 3 [Eight months later]
Admitted in great pain. Sweating profusely. We talked about her reasons for not having chemotherapy. She believes that the quality of her life is already poor and that it would reduce it further. Talked about death and she said that she was not afraid.
　　I taught her to breathe out in the face of panic; she did so and the sweating stopped as she calmed down.

Visit 4 [Fifteen days later]
Her colour is good but she says her pain is excessive. She asked me for a tape, which I provided.

Visit 5 [Three days later]
Great improvement; says that the tape is of considerable help. Asked for more tapes.

Visit 6 [Two days later]
Pain now relieved, looks totally different, and says that she is very grateful. Discharged home next day, I hear that she has been well and pain-free since.

Mrs R...
Diagnosis: Uncontrolled vomiting
[Referred by doctor to control vomiting]

Visit 1
Relaxed well, vomiting controlled.

Visit 2 [Next day]
Very jaundiced and feeling depressed, but relaxed well, no vomiting.

Visit 3 [Nine days later]
Very droopy and depressed; relaxed surprisingly well. Comfortable.

Visit 4 [Five days later]
Vomiting badly again. Relaxed her and it stopped. Colour improved and she said that she felt better.

Visit 5 [Next day]
In pain. Long talk about worries and aims. Has decided to give up work and enjoy her life. Relaxed well and pain went. Chemotherapy was started and she was unafraid. Good session.

Visit 6 [Next day]
Sleepy but much happier. No problems with chemotherapy.

Visit 7 [Next day]
About to vomit as I arrived, but she controlled it with relaxation.

Visit 8 [Next day]
Grateful for learning the method – 'Everyone says relax and fight but no one tells you how.'

Visit 9 [Three days later]
Has been home for the weekend and enjoyed herself. Eating well.

Visit 10 [Next day]
Did not mention relaxation on the ward round. Can I assume that it is no longer important to her? Discharged home.

Visit 11 [Two months later – re-admitted]
Referred by her doctor. She has regressed and is vomiting again. Relaxed well and it stopped.

Visit 12 [Two days later]
Using relaxation herself to control vomiting. Discharged home.

Visit 13 [Three weeks later – re-admitted]
More chemotherapy. Using relaxation well to control vomiting.

Mr F...
Diagnosis: Carcinoma of the bronchus. Has learning difficulties

Mr F... is used to being a very active man but finds that he has nothing to do to pass the time in hospital. I am teaching him to breathe gently and to move more easily so that it requires less effort. Says that he understands that he is dying and that he accepts this, and that learning relaxation gives him something positive to do which eases his symptoms.

Test cases

by Carol Horrigan

When I was asked to edit Ursula Fleming's writings, I decided to use the technique with some of the patients who were already learning relaxation with me. They were using basic tense–relax techniques, visualization methods including Simonton's method, Chakra and colour work, meditation and differing levels of altered states, from simple guided imagery to full hypnosis. I also used adjuncts including music and art, and olfactory (aromatherapy), and tactile input into combined methods.

Other patients who tried the Fleming method were using relaxation for the first time. I was therefore able to gain a cross-section of views of both its effects and its efficacy.

Some of these patients' profiles are presented here, with the results they achieved and their own impressions. All the patients gave permission for their cases to be included, but I have changed some identifying characteristics to maintain confidentiality.

As with Ursula's patients, the broad spectrum of problems helped by the Fleming Method is demonstrated. I too see many patients with cancer, and now also HIV-related illness. As their symptoms and problems are almost identical, I have also included case histories from other departments and clinics.

Patrick, aged 53
Presenting problem: Transient high blood pressure during emigration medical procedure

This patient had attended the designated doctor for a medical examination during emigration procedure. Previously, his blood pressure was within normal limits for his age but the recent pressure of work, and the process of emigration had begun to cause him stress and when he attended for the medical, his blood pressure was raised according to the criteria set by the emigration department. This meant that he was at risk of being refused permission to emigrate. The doctor was sympathetic and because he felt that it was a transient problem, he suggested that Patrick take a short break and re-attend for examination.

Patrick had never used relaxation before. He completed Lesson 1, and when I checked his blood pressure at the end of the session it was within the required parameters. His busy schedule prevented him from taking any more sessions but he felt confident, so he re-attended for medical, implemented the technique and was accepted for emigration.

Ishbel, aged 29
Presenting problem: Termination of pregnancy

Ishbel had been learning different methods of relaxation with me to control attacks of urticaria when she found that she was pregnant. Because she has congenital heart defects she was advised to terminate the pregnancy. Naturally she was distressed and contacted me to see if I could help her through the ordeal that lay ahead.

She attended for five sessions and found that by using the Fleming Method she was able to remain calm throughout her admission to hospital and could relax before and after the operation. Ishbel has been able to compare the method with the others that she has experienced and now prefers to use it for any stressful situation, although she still uses guided imagery and Chakra work for daily relaxation.

Joe, aged 45
Presenting problem: Bereavement following the traumatic death of a friend

Joe had always believed in the power of the mind and had used other complementary therapies for physical problems such as sciatica and hay fever. He had not used any self-help techniques before, always preferring to use a therapist for massage or osteopathy.

The death of Joe's friend in a train crash had left him feeling numbed but unable to release his grief. He said that he felt he wanted to scream and could feel pressure behind his eyes and in his head.

He attended for two sessions on consecutive days, and he completed lessons 1 and 2. After the first session he was more relaxed but still felt the need to cry, but the second session was instrumental in helping him to give vent to his feelings. That night he cried, and was angry by turns. Another friend stayed with him throughout and when I saw him next, Joe described his experience as 'cleansing'.

Grace, aged 27
Presenting problem: Irritable bowel syndrome

Newly diagnosed and frustrated by the fact that there was no 'simple pill' to help her discomfort, Grace was willing to try relaxation. She had been to yoga classes and had some idea of relaxation as the class leader always ended the session with a guided imagery session.

Grace attended weekly for twelve weeks. She completed all the lessons except those which included lying on the broomstick because she was already experiencing quite severe pain, and some lessons she repeated more than once.

From the first lesson she reported a reduction in pain, but she continued to attend because she wanted to be able to use the method for other stressful situations, thereby preventing the build-up of tension which exacerbates irritable bowel disease. By the end of the series of lessons Grace was symptom-free, and said that she felt much more 'in control of my life'.

Mandy, aged 31
Presenting problem: Depression and loss of appetite following enforced redundancy

Mandy had been employed in a very interesting job which also paid a high salary. When her company decided to reduce its workforce, she was made redundant as one of the people who had been in post for the shortest time; her employer had told her that the quality of her work had not been in question.

It did not alter the fact that Mandy had no income to maintain the lifestyle that she had enjoyed, and when she could not find another similar job, her savings were gradually used, until finally she had to sell her home in London and move back to her parents who lived in the country. She found the loss of independence intolerable, and began eating less and less so that she could have money available for travelling to be with her friends. Mandy did not find eating less a problem, she had always been careful with her diet in order to maintain a fashionably slender figure. When she came to see me she was worried. She now found that even the thought of food made her nauseous and both she and her family were alarmed at her low weight. She felt that if she could get rid of the tension in her abdomen, then she would want to eat again.

Mandy completed the lessons on relaxation, breathing, walking and seeing. She enjoyed the sensation of being in control again, and of being aware of her body. She remained unemployed for some time, but was able to be content living back in the country. She did not regain her weight but has not continued to lose more. The reactive mood swings continue, but she says that they are diminishing in both intensity and frequency.

James, aged 25
Presenting problem: Panic attacks when studying and taking examinations

There seemed to be no logical reason why James should suddenly have panic attacks at university. He had been an 'A' grade student at school and had entered the degree course of his choice without hindrance. When he came to ask if relaxation could help him, I met a young man who was showing all the signs of extreme agitation. He could not hold eye contact, was fidgeting in his chair, and constantly picking at his clothes or running his fingers through his hair. He told me how the panic attacks affected him with sweating, dry mouth and hyperventilation so severe that on one occasion he had lost consciousness. Fortunately he had been with a friend who was a medical student and he had known how to care for James. He claimed that he was aware of his heart beating rapidly. This had concerned him because he was physically very fit, participating in several sports regularly, and he knew that his normal standing pulse was low and steady. The panic attacks would most often begin when he tried to study after lectures.

James learned Lessons 1 and 2 and how to breathe lying down and sitting in a chair. At the end of session one, he said that he could feel a sensation of running water coursing through his body, where before it had seemed solid and 'blocked'. He started to control his panic from Lesson 1, even before he learned the lessons on breathing. By using his centre of stillness to calm his pulse rate and relax his extremities, he was able to control the attacks and find a sense of peace which enabled him to study.

In due course James was able to be relaxed enough to analyse why he had experienced the problems in the first place. He now realizes that he was simply worried that he would not be able to maintain his high standards and that he would be a disappointment to his parents if he failed to get a first class honours degree – a natural, and commonplace problem for university students. If he had not learned to relax, he may have done just that.

Carolynne, aged 18
Presenting problem: Bereavement stress

As a student nurse, Carolynne had already witnessed the death of patients, but when her grandmother died at home she was overcome with grief. She returned to her studies and her work, but felt isolated from her family for whom this had been the most recent of several deaths. Carolynne was not able to talk about her feelings at our first meeting, but gradually, by using relaxation, she was able to express her grief and deal with it. She thought that her reactions were extreme and, as many nurses do, believed that she should 'control herself' and that she was over-reacting to the situation. Using the breathing sessions enabled her to deal with her sighs and overbreathing, as these, she felt, were outward signs of lack of control.

Helen, aged 19
Presenting problem: Stress related to her younger sister's illness

When Helen first came to see me she simply asked me to teach her relaxation because she was working in a stressful job and she thought that it might help. Her body language told another story, but at a first meeting I could only observe and wait for her to offer information. We began using the method, and she was responding well. She had some experience of using relaxation techniques but did not define what they were. This information was given at the end of the first session, when she was describing her reactions and comparing them with sessions that she had attended on meditation and guided imagery.

The actual reason for Helen seeking relaxation lessons emerged in visit number three. Her younger sister was desperately ill with a rare and debilitating neurological disease. The sadness of her plight and the effect that it was having on the whole family was understandable, but Helen had hoped that she could have been stronger for their mother. The realization that she was not coping had brought her to see me.

Helen continued to visit me for several months, using Lessons 1 and 2 alternately. This was her choice, and she was successful in that she was able to cope both at work and at home when she was feeling stressed.

Terese, aged 31
Presenting problem: Chronic fatigue syndrome

Referred by her doctor, Terese was taking high doses of tranquillizers, a result of being diagnosed as having 'myalgic encephalomyelitis' (ME) more than ten years ago. At that time it was often viewed as a psychiatric problem, and patients were prescribed mood-altering drugs because there was simply nothing else to offer them. They did not have a recognizable psychiatric syndrome, but the many and often bizarre combinations of symptoms that patients listed (often up to sixty in number during the course of the disease process), seemed to indicate some form of psychosomatic disorder. Tranquillizers were therefore used to ease their apparent, but now known to be reactive, depression. The syndrome would follow in the wake of a simple viral infection, making life intolerable, as even the slightest effort would leave sufferers debilitated for hours after they had completed a simple task.

This was the situation that Terese found herself in, and now that she was considerably improved, with most of her physical symptoms subsiding or under control, she was looking forward to discontinuing taking medication.

She learned relaxation, and the seeing exercises, followed by the breathing exercises. She pronounced them a great success, saying that they made her feel 'refreshed and able to cope'.

Morgan, aged 45
Presenting problem: Chronic fatigue syndrome

Referred by his Consultant, Morgan had been through the worst of the experience of this syndrome, which has attracted much defamatory media attention and yet can be devastating for the sufferers. Morgan's problems had begun following an acute gastrointestinal upset. The 'flu-like symptoms that followed were to last for almost eight years. In that time he had been unable to work and had consequently lost his job in one of the major service industries. His remaining problems now consisted of abdominal pain after meals, sensitivity to many common and staple foods such as wheat and potatoes and also to stimulants, including coffee and tea.

I was requested to help him relax before he embarked upon a new career that required him to retrain, following a course of study including practical skills that would take him four years to complete.

Morgan was a very willing student and he decided to try to complete as many of the Fleming Method lessons as he could. He was able to experience them all except balancing the stick – this being impracticable in the small clinic room where we had our sessions. He found the method very effective in helping him to relax. The pain after meals receded and he felt he could look forward to his new career.

Christine, aged 23
Presenting problem: Psoriasis

Christine had tried several orthodox and complementary therapies for the relief of her symptoms and the accompanying distress of psoriasis. She had a high pressure job and could always assess when she would have a new patch appear in relation to the level of stress that she encountered on a daily basis.

At her first attempt at relaxing used the Fleming Method she could feel a difference in effect compared to other relaxation methods that she had tried. By the end of the second session she was already seeing a difference in the patches and in her response to the stressors which caused them.

Hilary, aged 32
Presenting problem: Thyrotoxicosis

The early symptoms of thyrotoxicosis are often subtle and difficult to define. Hilary just knew that she felt 'odd', 'not her usual self' and that her pulse was unusually fast – so fast that she was aware of it even when she was going to sleep. She had been seeing me for stress reduction sessions and we had tried several different approaches. When her diagnosis was confirmed it did not surprise me. Each time she had visited, the method chosen would work for a few hours and bring her some relief, but by the time I saw her the next week, she would be just the same as before.

We started to use the Fleming Method during the week of her diagnosis, when the Consultant told her that the orthodox treatment he had prescribed would take some time to be effective. She liked the feeling that the method brought her and was able to use it to help her relax at different points in the day until her medication began to be effective. She found that although her heart rate was still rapid, it did not make her feel stressed as before.

Pippa, aged 20
Presenting problem: Pre-menstrual syndrome

Pippa had 'always' experienced some discomfort prior to and during menstruation. Many women do have a difficult time when they menstruate but it is often due to the anticipated fear of pain rather than actual physiological disturbance. As Ursula Fleming describes, it can create a spiral of tension and pain which has to be broken.

Pippa had used many types of powerful and thoroughly unsuitable analgesics to no avail. Some she had obtained on prescription from her doctor, others she had bought in the local chemist. She often self-administered almost lethal cocktails of the two with the added danger of alcohol, in the mistaken belief that 'more is better'. They did not work.

When I explained about the Fleming Method I thought at first that she might reject the idea as she was so used to taking medication. Following her first two sessions she phoned to tell me that she had been practising each day and actually forgot when she was due to menstruate and so was surprised to find that the erstwhile dreaded event was upon her without her realizing it!

Joanne, aged 45
Presenting problem: Stress due to difficult neighbours

This patient was referred to me by her doctor because she had requested tranquillizers for what he considered to be an unsuitable reason. When dealing with stress, the best solution is to remove or minimize the stressor; sadly, unreasonably noisy neighbours cannot be removed or minimized easily.

At first Joanne thought the whole idea ludicrous. How could she reduce her stress when it was someone else who was creating it? Being a reasonable person meant that she was at least willing to give it a try. It took about six sessions, but eventually she had to admit that she was now able to get to sleep and stay asleep by using the method. I agreed with her that she should not have to resort to implementing any kind of counteraction against her surroundings simply to get some sleep, but life is a series of compromises and, rather than have insomnia, a few moments of practising a relaxation method was a small price to pay.

John, aged 20
Presenting problem: Sickle cell disease pain

John had been having massage, aromatherapy and healing to help him with the pain in his knees and hips. He used orthodox medication too but was keen to try methods that did not include the use of drugs. Many situations would trigger an attack, but he could never predict when it would happen and he was looking for something which would give him control under different circumstances.

He was already in pain and so we used only the relaxation and breathing lessons. The breathing lessons were important as patients in pain often breathe in an erratic fashion as the pain ebbs and flows and as they move around to avoid the pain. The excruciating pain of sickle cell disease is usually only countered by strong narcotic agents. For John, the effect of using the Fleming Method was not to eradicate the pain but to make it bearable, and to give him some respite when it returned between doses of medication.

Prudence, aged 34
Presenting problem: Insomnia

Prudence had been suffering from difficulties in sleeping for eight months when she was referred by her doctor for relaxation. As usual, I discussed with her the varied methods that could be used and she tried Reflex Therapy and Therapeutic Touch before embarking upon the Fleming Method.

Every night when she went to bed, she would recall all of her day's activities and critically analyse them. This can be a useful habit to adopt, but is best carried out before going to bed, having put all of the 'problems' to bed first. By doing it her way, Prudence was creating more stress as she tried to devise problem-solving plans whilst she should have been winding down before going to sleep.

She found that 'letting go' was the secret to her success. After learning to use the Fleming Method she could go to sleep 'in the moment'. With the method she had been able to 'let go' of her stressors and by doing so had released all the thoughts of past and future which had caused her insomnia.

Kirsty, aged 33
Presenting problem: Habitual abortion (miscarriage) stress

To experience the loss of one baby is sad, but to have it happen five times in as many years had left Kirsty not only with a feeling of sadness once more, but also with resentment and anger. She was worried that soon she would be too old to keep trying and that her dream of being a mother would be lost.

She was constantly thinking of only one subject and would torment herself by visiting shops that sold baby clothes and equipment, planning what she would choose for the new arrival when the day came.

We decided to work on her centre of stillness and to help her to let go of her repeating one-track thoughts. She also found herself heaving great sighs, which would accompany overwhelming feelings of regret. For this we used the breathing exercises.

Kirsty came to see me regularly and we would use the lessons each time as she decided she needed them, sometimes using part of one and part of another. After three months she was able to have whole days without thinking about babies at all, or if she did, then she would be able to be rational about it and put the thoughts to one side. She had learned to let go.

George, aged 39
Presenting problem: Stress at work and insomnia

Executive stress is not a myth, and it was happening to George. At a time when he would have preferred to be spending time with his growing family, George was working longer hours, travelling abroad more for his company and worrying each day that he might one day be made redundant in a company 'rationalization of staff'.

Consequently he was suffering from unexplained aches and pains, having difficulty getting to sleep at night and waking early in the morning with thoughts of work scurrying around in his mind. He had been to see his GP because he thought that he might have an organic problem. He was reassured that he was fit, and indeed he was. He played squash or went swimming at lunchtime, and had relinquished the car for a walk to and from the station each day.

Not sure about the efficacy of self-help techniques, George was sceptical about his abilities to use the method. To his scientific mind, it appeared far too simple to be a realistic answer. Also he confessed that he would far rather take a tablet – 'so much more logical, and quick too!' He had difficulty accepting that it was up to him to help himself, he had always relied on 'experts' before when he had health problems.

We talked about becoming an 'expert' and diagnosing and solving our own problems. He was able to use the method well, and could release the tension in his neck, relax to go to sleep and stay asleep for a normal amount of time, but it took him a long time to 'do it himself' and to stop feeling that it was more 'scientific' to pay for outside support.

Sandra, aged 29
Presenting problem: Post-diagnosis stress

It was following a routine cervical smear test that Sandra was found to have early carcinoma. The diagnosis and the fact that she might not be able to have children following surgery was the cause of her stress. She was due to be admitted within the next three weeks, but was unable to continue working as she could not control her emotions. She would suddenly find herself crying or losing concentration.

A friend recommended that she try relaxation and give up work for a while until her health improved.

Sandra came to see me three times and was an excellent student. She was very pleased with the results that she could achieve by using the method. Her friend's advice was accepted and she spent her time before the operation in concentrating on the positive and 'being in the moment'. Not looking backward or forward enabled her to stabilize her thoughts. The operation was a success and her follow-up showed no recurrence. She continues to live 'in the moment' enjoying her good health. When her Consultant gives her approval to become pregnant, then she will begin to look forward again.

Rose, aged 74
Presenting problem: Neck pain

Rose has been suffering from neck pain for more than fifty years. It began when she was pregnant for the first time at the age of twenty-two. Various diagnoses have been given to her down the years and she has never found anything but transient relief from analgesics, support collars, physiotherapy, massage and several other therapies. She has developed what Ursula would describe as a spiral of pain and tension. Afraid to let go of the tension in case it causes any more pain, Rose had developed a rigidity in her neck muscles which she now believed to be permanent. After only one session, using the head and neck release exercise, she could feel a difference and a sense of release in the muscles, and could immediately move her head further than she had for as long as she could remember. She continues to practise – 'when she remembers', because she is busy doing things that she hasn't dared to do for years.

Elspeth, aged 25
Presenting problem: Fear of surgery

When Elspeth was told that she needed major surgery to re-shape her bladder she at first refused to consider the idea. Repeated bouts of painful cystitis had brought her to the urology clinic, and investigations had shown up the problem. An overlarge bladder with constant retention of urine was the culprit. Elspeth was horrified, both at the thought of her body being so 'deformed' and at the thought of a major operation.

Her Consultant referred her to me for relaxation as he considered it imperative for her future health that Elspeth have the operation as soon as possible. In discussion, she revealed her fear of further pain, although she knew that it would in fact cure the pain that she was experiencing so frequently.

She undertook to try out lying and standing on a stick, and so she embarked upon an intensive training in relaxation. She came every other day, starting from scratch and learning everything she could about pain control. Before she was admitted for surgery, she experienced yet another episode of cystitis and was able to cope with the pain. She used relaxation before her pre-med and when she recovered from the anaesthetic. Her rapid recovery was remarked upon by all the nursing and medical staff, and when I saw her again I asked her how she had coped. 'It was a breeze!' she replied.

Alice, aged 10
Presenting problem: Eczema
[Editor's note: Eczema often occurs in children (and adults) when their emotional support system is under stress.]

Alice has been coming to see me since she was three years old; she has tried many different complementary therapies for the eczema that has plagued her from then. Each therapy would work for a while, but because her family situation is very unstable eventually the blisters and cracks would return and she would again be unable to carry out many everyday tasks without difficulty. Her greatest distress was being called names at school and finding that other children did not want to hold her hand when they had to walk in twos.

For three years she has been quite successful using guided imagery to 'cool' her hands when they itch, but using the Fleming Method to bring all the itching to her 'centre of stillness' and to hold on to that thought 'in the moment', she has not had an outbreak for six months. She is excited about what she can do and is constantly showing people her now beautifully soft hands.

Jane, aged 40
Asthma

Jane explained her life as 'complicated and stressful'. She holds a very responsible position in local government and manages to juggle the demands of her private and public life by working long hours with little time to think about her own well-being. Consequently, the asthma attacks which she had experienced since childhood had recently become more frequent and more prolonged, requiring her to take medication every day. She found that she had difficulties breathing in meetings, when taking stressful phone calls and again when she arrived home to face the different needs of her family.

We began by using Lessons 1 and 2 to begin to allow her time for herself, and she would practise them in the morning and again in the evening before going to bed. These were followed by breathing and posture exercises (Lessons 7 and 8) and seeing and walking in a relaxed way (Lessons 10 and 11).

After the first two lessons Jane was pleased with her ability to control her fear of the possibility of an attack. The breathing lessons helped particularly with her poor breathing patterns when answering the phone. The seeing and walking lessons were included because, in discussion with Jane about finding time for herself in her busy days, she decided that she could use the skills that those lessons would give her to maintain the relaxation in her daily activities.

Jane was very impressed by her own abilities to cope with her breathing during her working day. The breathing lessons had completely eradicated the need for her to use medication at the office. She has almost totally discontinued its use at home. The only time she finds it is necessary to use an inhaler is if the weather is very cold or she does not have time to do her exercises before she has to deal with the breakfast-time rush of family needs.

Epilogue

by Anne Fleming

Ursula Fleming used her relaxation method to help many women through childbirth. No record has been found of any of these sessions. However, after Ursula's death I came across *The Squire*, a novel by Enid Bagnold published in 1938, when Ursula was eight years old. To my amazement I found in this book a description of a woman in labour using the same method for coping with pain taught by Ursula (i.e. the method of accepting the pain without reservation, treating it not as pain but as sensation).

Ursula never read the book, nor did she meet Enid Bagnold. Had she known of the passage in *The Squire*, I am sure she would immediately have sought the author out. It is possible that Enid Bagnold learned of the method through Ursula's teacher Gertrude Heller, or she may have learnt it from a teacher of meditation or yoga, both of which had become more accessible in the West by then, but it is much more likely that she worked it out for herself from her own experience of childbirth. It is a powerful description of an intelligent and strong-minded woman conquering what has been described as the worst pain of all by questioning the usual attitude to pain.

The italics are mine: their purpose is to point out the most marked similarities with Ursula's teaching.

'Is this really pain or is it an extraordinary sensation?'

'What's the difference? Pain is but a branch of sensation. *Perhaps childbirth turns into pain only when it is fought and resisted?* I'm aching, I'm restless. I can't tell you how but there comes a time after the first pains have passed when you swim down a silver river running like a torrent with the convulsive corkscrew movements of a great fish, threshing from its neck to its tail. And if you can marry the movements, go with them, turn like a screw in the river and swim on, then the pain, then I believe *the pain – becomes a flame that doesn't burn you.'*

'Awful,' said Caroline, shuddering.

'It's not awful. The thing's progressive. And when you are right in the river, to marry the pain requires tremendous determination and will and self-belief. *You have to rush ahead into it and not pull back against it.'* ...

The Birth

Her mind went down and lived in her body, ran out of her brain and lived in her flesh. She had eyes and nose and ears and senses in her body, living like a spiny woodlouse doubled like a ball, having no beginning and no end ...

Now the first twisting spate of pain began. Swim then, swim with it for your life! *If you resist, horror and impediment! If you swim, not pain but sensation!* Who knows the heart of pain, the silver whistling hub of pain, the central bellows of childbirth which expels one being from another? None knows it who, in disbelief and dread, has drawn back to the periphery, contradicting the will of pain, braking against inexorable movements. Keep abreast of it, rush together, you and the violence that is also you! Wild movements, hallucinated swimming! *Other things exist than pain!*

It is hard to gauge pain. By her movements, by her exclamations she would have struck horror into anyone other than her doctor and her midwife. She would have seemed tortured, tossing, crying, muttering, grunting. She was not unconscious, but she had left external life. She was blind and deaf to world surface. Every sense she had was down in earth to which she belonged, fighting to maintain a hold on the pain, to keep pace with it, *not to take an ounce of will from her assent to its passage.*

The Squire, by Enid Bagnold, published by William Heinemann, 1938

References and further reading

Abromowitz, S.I., and Weiselberg, N. (1978) Reaction to relaxation and desensitization outcome: five angry treatment failures. *American Journal of Psychiatry,* **135**, 1418–19

Baker, G.H. (1978) Psychological factors and immunity. *Journal of Psychosomatic Research,* **31**, 1–10

Beck, A.T. (1976) *Cognitive Therapy and the Emotional Disorders*, New York, International Universities Press

Beck, A.T. (1984) Cognitive approaches to stress management. In *Principles and Practice of Stress Management* (eds R.L. Woolfolk and P.M. Lehrer), New York, Guilford Press

Benson, H. (1976) *The Relaxation Response*, London, Collins

Bernstein, D.A. and Borkovec, T.D. (1973) *Progressive Relaxation Training: a Manual for the Helping Professions*, Champaign, Ill, Research Press

Bernstein, D.A. and Given, B.A. (1984) Progressive relaxation: abbreviated methods. In *Principles and Practice of Stress Management* (eds R.L. Woolfolk and P.M. Lehrer), New York, Guilford Press

Bloom, L.J. and Gonzales, A.M. (1981) Anxiety management with schizophrenic outpatients. *Journal of Clinical Psychology,* **38**, 280–85

Bond, M. (1986) *Stress and Self-Awareness: a Guide for Nurses*, Oxford, Butterworth-Heinemann

Borkovec, T.D. and Sides, J.K. (1979) Critical procedural variables related to the physiological effects of progressive relaxation: a review. *Behaviour Research and Therapy,* **17**, 119–25

Burke, J.B. (1989) An investigation of the effects of a stress management program on reported levels of stress/anxiety and time perception in registered nurses in the workplace. DNsc. Thesis, Boston University

Burnard, P. (1992) *Know Yourself! Self-awareness Activities for Nurses*, London, Scutari Press

Carty, J.L. (1990) Relaxation with imagery: an adjunctive treatment for nausea or vomiting. DNSc. Thesis, The Catholic University of America

Charlesworth, E.A. and Nathan, R.G. (1984) *Stress Management*, New York, Atheneum

Cobb, S.C. (1984) Teaching relaxation techniques to cancer patients. *Cancer Nursing,* **7** (2), 156–61

Cohen, F. (1980) Postsurgical pain relief: patients' status and nurses' medication choices. *Pain,* **9**, 265–74

Cox, T. (1978) *Stress*, London, Macmillan

Cox, T. and Mackay, C.J. (1976) *A psychological model of occupational stress. (Mental Health in Industry)* London, The Medical Research Council

Davidson, R.J. and Schwartz, G.E. (1976) The psychobiology of relaxation and related states: a multiprocess theory. In *Behaviour Control and Modification of Physiological Activity* (ed. D.I. Mostofky), Englewood Cliffs, NJ, Prentice-Hall

Davis, M., Eschelman, E. and McKay, M. (1988) *The Relaxation and Stress Reduction Workbook*, 3rd Edn., Oakland, CA, New Harbinger

Davis, P. (ed.) (1993) *Orthopaedic Nursing*, London, Heinemann

Deatrick, J.A. (1990) Developing self-regulation in adolescents with chronic conditions. *Holistic Nursing Practice*, **5** (1), 17–22

Donovan, M.I. (1980) Relaxation with guided imagery: a useful technique. *Cancer Nursing*, **3**, 27–32

Ellis, A. (1962) *Reason and Emotion in Psychotherapy*, New York, Lyle Stuart

Erseck, M. (1986) Stress and cancer: elusive connections. *Oncology Nursing Forum*, **13**, 49–56

Everly, G.S. and Rosenfeld, R. (1981) *The Nature and Treatment of the Stress Response*, New York, Plenum Press

Fanning, P. (1988) *Visualisation for Change*, Oakland, CA, New Harbinger

Fisher, E. (1988) Early experiences of a multidisciplinary pain management programme. *Holistic Medicine*, **3**, 47–56

Fleming, U. (1985) Relaxation therapy for far-advanced cancer. *The Practitioner*, **229**, 471–5

Fleming, U. (1988) Relaxation as a means of pain control. *Journal of Orthopaedic Medicine*, No.1, 21–23

Fleming, U. (1990) *Grasping the Nettle*, London, Collins/Fount

Fleming, U. (1995) *Meister Eckhart: The Man From Whom God Hid Nothing*, 2nd edn, Leominster, Gracewing/Fowler Wright Books

Fleming, U. (1995) *The Desert and the Marketplace: Writings, Letters, Journals* (ed. A. Fleming), Leominster, Gracewing/Fowler Wright Books

Frank, J.M. (1985) The effects of music therapy and guided visual imagery on chemotherapy-induced nausea and vomiting. *Oncology Nursing Forum*, **12** (5), 47–52

Gardner, W.N. and Bass, C. (1989) Hyperventilation in clinical practice. *British Journal of Hospital Medicine*, **41**, 73–81

Geden, E.A. (1989) Effects of music and imagery on psychologic self-report of labour pain. *Nursing Research*, **38** (1), 37–41

Giddens, A. (1979) *Central Problems in Social Theory*, London, Macmillan

Goldfreid, M.R. (1971) Effectiveness of relaxation as a coping skill. *Journal of Abnormal Psychology*, **83** (4), 348–355

Hamilton-Birney, M. (1991) Psychoneuroimmunology: A holistic framework for the study of stress and illness. *Holistic Nursing Practice*, **5** (4), 32–38

Hase, S. and Douglas, A. (1987) Effects of relaxation training on recovery from myocardial infarction. *Australian Journal of Advanced Nursing*, **5** (11), 18–27

Heide, F.J. and Borkovec, T.D. (1984) Relaxation-induced anxiety: mechanisms and theoretical implications. *Behaviour Research and Therapy*, **22**, 1–12

Hillenberg, J.B. and Collins, F.L. (1983) The importance of home practice for progressive relaxation training. *Behaviour Research and Training*, **21**, 633–42

Hillhouse, J. and Adler, C. (1991) Stress, health and immunity: a review of the literature and implications for the nursing profession. *Holistic Nursing Practice*, **5** (4), 22–31

Holden-Lund, C. (1988) Effects of guided imagery on surgical stress and wound healing. *Research in Nursing and Health*, **11** (4), 235–244

Holmes, S. (1991) Clinical leadership: a role for the advanced practitioner. *Advances in Health and Nursing*, **1** (3), 3–20

Holmes, S. and Dickerson, J.W.T. (1991) The quality of life: Design and evaluation of a self-assessment instrument for use with cancer patients. *International Journal of Nursing Studies*, **1** (24), 15–24

Hough, A. (1991) *Physiotherapy in Respiratory Care: a Problem-Solving Approach*, London, Chapman and Hall

Houldin, A.D., Lev, E., Prystowsky, M.B. *et al.* (1991) Psychoneuroimmunology: a review of the literature. *Holistic Nursing Practice*, **5** (4), 10–21

Hutchinson, M. (1984) *The Book of Floating*, New York, William Morrow

Innocenti, D.M. (1983) Chronic hyperventilation syndrome, in *Cash's Textbook of Chest Heart and Vascular Disorders for Physiotherapists*, 3rd edn (ed. P.A. Downie), London, Faber & Faber

Jackson, A. (1990) *Stress control through self-hypnosis*, London, Piatkus

Jacobson, E. (1938) *Progressive Relaxation*, 2nd edn, Chicago, University of Chicago Press

Jacobson, E. (1964) *Anxiety and Tension Control*, Philadelphia, J.B. Lippincott

Jacobson, E. (1976) *You Must Relax*, London, Souvenir Press

Karle, H. and Boyse, J. (1985) *Hypnotherapy*, London, Free Association Books

Kelly, G.A. (1955) *The Psychology of Personal Constructs*, New York, Norton

Kelly, J.O. (1984) Standards of clinical nursing practice for leukaemia: Anorexia, Nausea, Vomiting and fluid volume deficit. *Cancer Nursing*, 62–66

Kermani, K.S. (1990) *Autogenic Training*, London, Souvenir Press

Kolcabar, K.Y. and Kolcabar, R.J. (1991) An analysis of the concept of comfort. *Journal of Advanced Nursing*, **16**, 1301–10

Kolkmeier, L.G. (1987) Relaxation – opening the door to change. In *Holistic Nursing* (eds B.M. Dossey *et al.*), Gaithersburg, Aspen Pub. Inc.

Kokoszka, A. (1992) Relaxation as an altered state of consciousness: a rationale for a general theory of relaxation. *International Journal of Psychosomatics*, **39**, 4–9

Lehrer, P.M. (1982) How to relax and how not to relax: a re-evaluation of the work of Edmund Jacobson. *Behaviour Research and Therapy*, **20**, 417–28

Lehrer, P.M. and Woolfolk, R.L. (1983) Are stress reduction techniques interchangeable or do they have specific effects? In *Stress Reduction Techniques* (eds R. L. Woolfolk and P. M. Lehrer), New York, Guilford Press

Lehrer, P.M., Batey, D.M. *et al.* (1988) The effect of repeated tense–release sequences on EMG and self-report of muscle tension: An evaluation of Jacobsonian and post-Jacobsonian assumptions about progressive relaxation. *Psychophysiology*, **25**, 562–567

Levin, R.F. *et al.* (1987) Nursing management of post-operative pain: use of relaxation techniques with cholecystomy patients. *Journal of Advanced Nursing*, **12**, 463–572

Lichstein, K.L. (1983) Ocular relaxation as a treatment for insomnia. *Behavioural Counselling and Community Interventions*, **3**, 178–85

Lichstein, K.L. (1988) *Clinical Relaxation Strategies*, New York, John Wiley

Leibeskind, J.C. and Melzack, R. (1987) The International Pain Foundation: Meeting a need for education in pain management (Editorial). *Pain*, **30**, 1–2

Looker, T. and Gregson, O. (1989) *Stresswise: a Practical Guide for Dealing with Stress*, London, Hodder & Stoughton

Lucic, K.S., Steffan, J.J., Harrigan, J.A. and Stubeing, R.C. (1991) Progressive relaxation training: muscle contractions before relaxation. *Behaviour Therapy*, **22**, 249–56

Marks, R.M. and Sachar, E.J. (1973) Undertreatment of medical patients with narcotic analgesics. *Annals of Internal Medicine*, **78**, 173–81

Markut, C.F. (1989) Effects of nonprocedural touch and relaxation training on the psychophysiological stress level of patients undergoing cardiac catheterisation. DNSc Thesis, The Catholic University of America

Mastenboek, I. and McGovern, L. (1991) The effectiveness of relaxation techniques on controlling chemotherapy induced nausea: a literature review. *Australian Occupational Therapy Journal*, **28**, 137–42

Mather, L. and Mackie, J. (1983) The incidence of postoperative pain in children. *Pain*, **15**, 271–82

McCaffrey, M. (1979) *Nursing Management of the Patient with Pain*, 2nd edn, Philadelphia, J. B. Lippincott

McCaffrey, M. (1983) *Nursing the Patient in Pain*, London, Harper & Rowe

McCaffrey, M. and Beeb, A. (1989) *Pain: a Clinical Manual for Nursing Practice*, St Louis, C.V. Mosby

McCormack, G.L. (1992) The therapeutic benefits of the relaxation response. *Occupational Therapy Practice*, **4**, 51–60

McGuigan, F.J. (1984) Progressive relaxation: origins, principles and clinical applications. In *Principles and Practice of Stress Management* (eds R.L. Woolfolk and P.M. Lehrer), New York, Guilford Press

Meichenbaum, D. and Cameron, R. (1983) Stress inoculation training. In *Stress Reduction and Prevention* (eds D. Meichenbaum and M. E. Jarenko), New York, Plenum Press

Melzack, R. and Wall, P.D. (1965) Pain Mechanisms: a new theory. *Science*, **150**, 971–979

Merskey, H., Albe-Fessard, D.G., Bonica, J. J. *et al.* (1979) Pain terms: a list with definitions and notes on usage. *Pain*, **6**, 249-52

Mitchell, L. (1987) *Simple Relaxation: the Mitchell Method for Easing Tension*, 2nd edn, London, John Murray

Mooney, K.H., Ferrell, B.R., Nail, L.M. *et al.* (1991) 1991 Oncology Nursing Society Research Priority Survey. *Oncology Nursing Forum*, **18** (8), 1381–1388

Moss, V. (1985) Beating the stress connection. *Association of Operating Room Nurses*, **41** (4), 720

Murphy, L.R. (1983) A comparison of relaxation methods for reducing stress in nursing personnel. *Human Factors*, **35** (4), 431

Nixon, P.G.F. (1988) Human functions and the heart. In *Changing Ideas in Health Care* (eds D. Seedhouse and A. Cribb), Chichester, John Wiley

Ost, L.G. (1987) Applied relaxation: description of a coping technique and review of controlled studies. *Behaviour Therapy and Treatment*, **25**, 397–407

Padilla, G.V. and Grant, M.M. (1985) Quality of care as a nursing outcome variable. *Advances in Nursing Science*, **8** (1), 45–60

Paul, G.L. (1969) Physiological effects of relaxation training and hypnotic suggestion. *Journal of Abnormal Psychology*, **74**, 425–37

Payne, R.A. (1989) Glad to be yourself: a course of practical relaxation and health education talks. *Physiotherapy*, **75**, 8–9

Peper, E. and Williams, E.A. (1981) *From the Inside Out*, New York, Plenum Press

Poppen, R. (1988) *Behavioural Relaxation Training and Assessment*, Oxford, Pergamon Press

Powell, T.J. and Enright, S.J. (1990) *Anxiety and Stress Management*, London, Routledge

Randolph, G.L., Price J.L. and Collins, J.R. (1986) The effects of symptoms in nurses. *Journal of Continuing Education*, **17** (2), 43

Redd, W.H. and Jacobsen, P.B. (1988) Emotions and cancer: new perspectives on an age old question. *Cancer*, **62**, 1871–9

Salkovskis, P.M. (1988) Hyperventilation and anxiety. *Current Opinion in Psychiatry*, **1**, 76–82

Schain, W. (1980) Patients' rights in decision making. *Cancer Nursing*, **3**, 1035–41

Schilling, D.J. and Poppen, R. (1983) Behavioural relaxation training and assessment. *Journal of Behaviour Therapy and Experimental Psychiatry*, **14** 99–107

Seers, K. (1989) Patients' perceptions of acute pain. In *Directions in Nursing Research: Ten Years of Progress at London University* (eds. J. Wilson-Barnett and S. Robinson), London, Scutari Press

Seyle, H. (1950) *The Physiology and Pathology of Exposure to Stress*, Montreal, Acta

Seyle, H. (1956) *The Stress of Life*, New York, McGraw Hill

Seyle, H. (1973) The evolution of the stress concept. *American Scientist*, **61**, 692–9

Seyle, H. (1974) *Stress without Distress*, Scarborough, New American Library of Canada

Sims, S.E.R. (1987) Relaxation training as a technique for helping patients cope with the experience of cancer: a selective review of the literature. *Journal of Advanced Nursing*, **12**, 583–91

Simonton, O.C., Matthews-Simonton, S. and Creighton, J.L. (1986) *Getting well again*, London, Bantam

Smith, P. (1992) *The Emotional Labour of Nursing*, London, Macmillan Education Ltd.

Snyder, M. (1985) *Independent Nursing Interventions*, New York, John Wiley

Spence, A.A. (1991) Pain after surgery. *Journal of Bone and Joint Surgery*, **73-B** (2), 189–90

Spiegel, D., Bloom, J.R., Kraemer, H.C. and Gottheil, E. (1989) Effect of psychosocial treatment on survival of patients with metastatic cancer. *Lancet*, **10** (2), 888–91

Stevens, J.O. (1971) *Awareness: Exploring, Experimenting, Experiencing*, Moab, Real People Press

Strongman, K.T. (1987) *The Psychology of Emotion*, Chichester, John Wiley

Titlebaum, H. (1988) Relaxation, in *Relaxation and Imagery: Tools for Therapeutic Communication and Intervention* (ed. R. P. Zahourek), Philadelphia, W. B. Saunders

Tschudin, V. (1991) *Beginning with Awareness: a Learners' Handbook*, Edinburgh, Churchill Livingstone

Van Nguyen, T. (1991) Mind, brain and immunity: a critical review. *Holistic Nursing Practice*, **5** (4), 1–9

Varrichio, C. (1990) The relevance of the quality of life to clinical nursing practice. *Seminars in Oncology Nursing*, **6** (4), 255–9

Vines, S.W. (1988) The therapeutics of guided imagery. *Holistic Nursing Practice*, **2** (3), 34–44

Walding, M.F. (1991) Pain, anxiety and powerlessness. *Journal of Advanced Nursing*, **16**, 388–97

Watson, M. (ed.) (1991) *Cancer Patient Nursing: Psychological Treatment Methods*, Cambridge, BSP Books and Cambridge University Press

Watt-Watson, J. (1987) Nurses' knowledge of pain issues: a survey. *Journal of Pain and Symptom Management*, **2**, 207–11

Weis, O.F., Sriwatanakul, K., Allozoa, I.I. *et al.* (1983) Attitudes of patients, house staff and nurses towards post-operative analgesic care. *Anaesthesia and Analgesia*, **62**, 70–4

Woolfolk, L.R. and Lehrer, P.M. (eds.) (1984) *Principles and Practice of Stress Management*, New York, Guilford Press

Index

Coventry University

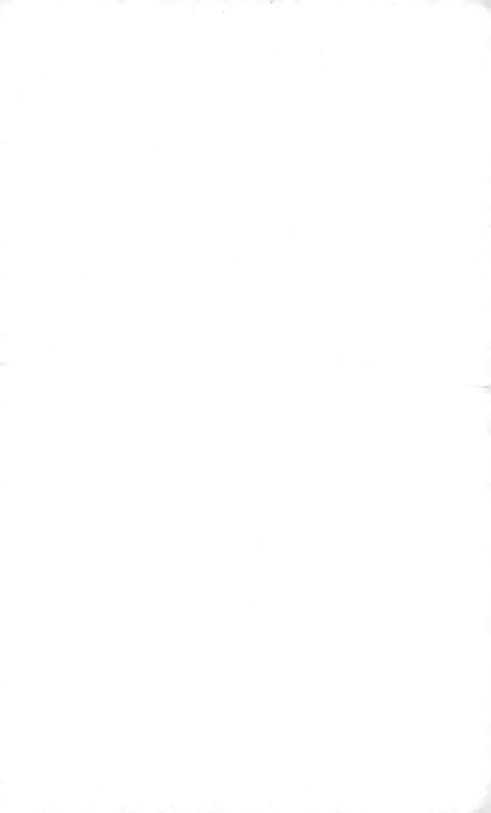